Dee Gano

D1109761

essentials
of dental radiography
for
dental assistants
and hygienists

Wolf R. de Lyre

Cerritos College

PRENTICE-HALL, INC., Englewood Cliffs, New Jersey

Library of Congress Cataloging in Publication Data

de Lyre, Wolf R. (date)
  Essentials of dental radiography for dental
assistants and hygienists.

  Includes bibliographical references.
  1. Teeth—Radiography. I. Title.
[DNLM: 1. Radiography, Dental. WN230 D367e]
RK309.D44   617.6'07'572   74-16170
ISBN 0-13-285684-0

© 1975 by Prentice-Hall, Inc.
Englewood Cliffs, New Jersey

All rights reserved. No part of this book
may be reproduced in any form or by any means
without permission in writing from the publisher.

10 9 8 7 6 5 4

Printed in the United States of America

PRENTICE-HALL INTERNATIONAL, INC., *London*
PRENTICE-HALL OF AUSTRALIA, PTY. LTD., *Sydney*
PRENTICE-HALL OF CANADA, LTD., *Toronto*
PRENTICE-HALL OF INDIA PRIVATE LIMITED, *New Delhi*
PRENTICE-HALL OF JAPAN, INC., *Tokyo*

contents

13
interproximal or bitewing examination   *168*

14
the occlusal examination   *178*

15
radiography for children   *187*

preface

Interest in dental radiography is at an all time high. Preventive radiation, which includes early detection of dental decay and periodontal lesions, is routinely practiced in most dental offices. Although this benefits the patient, it also exposes both patient and operator to x-radiation and any exposure is accompanied by a degree of risk to the cell structures.

In recognition of this, radiation safety legislation has been passed in many states and be being considered in others. In California, for example, users of radiation must first pass a safety examination. This law applies to licensed dentists and dental hygienists as well as unlicensed personnel. Students and trainees must practice with phantoms (dexters) or skulls and cannot make patient exposures before receiving the safety certificate.

Expanded duties for assistants and hygienists, continuing education requirements for dental and dental hygiene license renewal, and formal training with mandatory certification or licensing for dental assistants are being considered by many state legislators. Dental radiography is stressed on state and national boards. In recent years, one third of the national dental assistant certification test has been devoted to radiography questions. Since the busy, modern dentist delegates all phases of radiography except making the final diagnosis to his auxiliaries, he is less inclined to hire untrained personnel.

The objective of this book is to present the essentials of efficiently and safely producing radiographs of diagnostic value. The initial chapters explain equipment operation, x-ray characteristics, technical aspects of radiation, hazards of uncontrolled use, and safety precautions. Next, film processing, identification, mounting, and preliminary interpretation are described, with special emphasis on recognition of anatomic landmarks, lesions, the appearance of restorations on the radiographs, and causes and corrections of technique errors. The later chapters describe the theory and technical application of the principal exposure techniques of interest to the radiographer. The next to last chapter is devoted to dental photography, considered by many dentists to be an adjunct to radiography. The final chapter stresses patient education. The future of our profession and the dental health of our patients depends on how well we as dentists, and our co-workers, the dental assistants and hygienists, communicate with our patients and advance the concept of preventive radiography.

While this book is primarily intended as a text for college dental assisting and dental hygiene classes, it may also serve as a handy review for dentists, dental hygienists, or other auxiliaries who must prepare for safety tests or continuing education requirements. Also the trainee or assistant who is unable to enroll in radiography courses may find it useful for self-study, especially if used in conjunction with the accompanying workbook that provides assignments ranging from simple to complex intraoral and extraoral exposures.

It is recognized that the background and experience of the reader will vary. Some will have completed many units of science; others none. Every effort has been made to keep the language and the explanations simple, while using professional terminology. Recognizing that many with minimal previous science training would be frustrated by the vast number of scientific and specialized terms, most terms are explained either as they occur or in the glossary.

This book does not pretend to present new knowledge or to be the source of detailed technical information but hopefully it does include the essentials required to make most common exposures and to pass the safety, certification, or board tests. Reference is made in various sections of the book to special reference texts that the reader should consult for specific details, and to the many publications that were used in preparing this book. In most instances, the techniques shown have been used many years and are common knowledge in radiography. All references are listed in the bibliography at the end of each chapter. The serious reader is encouraged to consult these fine works. Many authors have permitted the use of materials or illustrations from their writings. These are all acknowledged as they appear.

It is virtually impossible to thank all the many professional friends and other persons who have become involved in the production of this book. In addition to the already mentioned authors, I thank Dr. Gerald Longhurst of UCLA and Dr. William J. Updegrave of Temple University for their valuable assistance in offering suggestions and correcting errors in the first draft of this manuscript. Credit also is deserved for the technical assistance given by Eastman Kodak, General Electric, and the Rinn Corporations, as well as other manufacturers that generously supplied materials and illustrations. Many of the radiographs were provided by professional friends, others by the radiography department of UCLA or by the McCormack X-Ray Laboratory. Their contributions are appreciated.

None of this would have been possible without the use of the excellent training facilities of Cerritos College and the encouragement received from Doris Sanson, division chairman, from Sonora Spencer who was instrumental in interesting me in teaching dental radiography, from my colleagues in the dental assisting and dental hygiene department, and from those wonderful dedicated students of Cerritos College who helped me to develop, test, and refine the workbook assignments and to eliminate unclear ideas or impractical assignments.

This acknowledgement would not be complete without my expression of gratitude to those who reviewed this book, Lucy Brajevich, Randall E. Culver, and H. M. Gagliardi, and to Barbara Archer and the excellent editorial and proof-reading staff of Prentice-Hall, Inc.

And finally, my sincerest gratitude to my wife, who has lived with this project since its inception five years ago, and has had a part in every page.

Wolf R. de Lyre

1

radiography
in dental practice

introduction

Modern dentistry is progressing so rapidly that changes in equipment and methods of practice are constantly taking place. One of these methods is radiography. Because correct diagnosis forms the basis for adequate dental treatment, the dentist requires radiographs of satisfactory quality. In recent years the use of radiography has become a routine procedure in the practice of dentistry.

As public demand for dental services increases, dentists are expanding the duties of their trained auxiliaries to include the exposure, processing, and mounting of x-ray films. The diagnosis of the radiographs is never done by the auxiliaries; that is the sole responsibility of the dentist. Although the laws vary from state to state, the authority to expose radiograph is either given or implied, provided these procedures are carried out under the dentist's supervision.

Good radiographs seldom happen by chance—they are the result of careful training and application of knowledge. All auxiliaries working with radiographic equipment should be thoroughly trained and versed in the theory of x-ray production, the operation of the x-ray unit, the various techniques commonly used to expose and process the films, as well as patient management and radiation safety procedures. Radiographs produced by good modern techniques allow the dentist to diagnose accurately. At the same time, they protect the patient and the dental auxiliary from receiving too much exposure to radiation. Both of these are important considerations.

discovery of the roentgen ray

The discovery of x-rays, unlike man's first steps on the moon, was not watched by millions of people. Only one person witnessed the event in a darkened room, but the words of Neil Armstrong about his Apollo mission that it was "one small step forward for man and a giant leap for mankind" can apply to this discovery as well. Professor Wilhelm Roentgen's experiment in Germany in 1895 produced a tremendous advance in science.

During an experiment with a low-pressure discharge tube covered with black paper, Professor Roentgen's curiosity was aroused when he observed that a fluorescent screen near the tube began to glow when the tube was activated. Examining this strange phenomenon further, he noticed that shadows could be cast on the screen by interposing objects between it and the tube. Further experimentation showed that such shadow images could be permanently recorded on photographic film. In the beginning Roentgen was uncertain of the nature of this invisible ray that he had accidentally discovered. When he later reported his findings at a scientific meeting he spoke of it as an "x-ray" because the symbol x represented the unknown. After his findings were reported and published, fellow scientists honored him be calling the invisible ray the *roentgen ray* and the image produced on photosensitive film a *roentgenograph*. Whether the image is called an x-ray picture, a roentgenograph, or a radiograph makes no difference—the terms are interchangeable. The patient is best acquainted with the word *x-ray*; the scientist and professional man generally prefer roentgenograph or radiograph. Because there is a basic similarity between a photographic negative and an x-ray film, and the x-ray closely resembles the radio wave, the prefix *radio* and the suffix *graphy* have been combined into radiograph. The latter term is gaining acceptance in professional offices because it is more descriptive than x-ray and easier to pronounce than roentgenograph.

early progress and development

Little of the progress achieved by medical and dental science would have been possible without *radiography*, which can be defined as the science or the process of generating and applying x-radiation to sensitized film for the purpose of making a shadow picture. A few weeks after Professor Roentgen announced his discovery, Dr. Otto Walkoff, a German physicist, exposed a prototype of a dental radiograph. It is believed that in 1896 Dr. William Rollins of Boston exposed the first dental radiograph in the United States. Although he wrote many scientific articles, Dr. Rollins remained a rather obscure figure. He was one of the first to alert the profession to the need for radiation hygiene and protection and is considered by many to be the father of the science of radiation protection. Unfortunately, his advice was not taken seriously by many of his fellow practitioners for a long time. Several years passed before the potential benefits and hazards of Professor Roentgen's discovery were fully appreciated.

Because x-rays are invisible, the pioneers in the field of radiography were not aware that exposure to them produced accumulations of radiation in the body and, therefore, could be dangerous to both patient and radiographer. When radiography was in its infancy, it was common practice for the dentist to help the patient hold the film in place while making the exposure; thus the dentist exposed himself needlessly to dangerous radiation. Frequent repetition of this practice endangered the dentist's health and occasionally led to permanent injury or death. Fortunately, although the hazards of prolonged exposure to radiation are not completely understood, we have learned how to reduce them drastically by proper use of safer x-ray machines. Placing a protective lead apron over the patient's lap makes him even safer, and the practice of having the radiographer stand behind structural or lead shielding affords him protection from stray, or secondary, radiation.

Today, when almost half of the radiation-producing equipment used in the United States is in dental offices, it is worth noting that as late as 1920 few hospitals and only the most progressive physicians and dentists possessed x-ray equipment. One of the earliest users, and a strong advocate of dental radiography in this country, was Dr. Edmund Kells of New Orleans. He made numerous presentations to organized dental groups and was instrumental in convincing many dentists that they should use dental radiography as a diagnostic tool. Unfortunately, he lost his life—as many other pioneers in radiography did—from excess radiation. At that time it was still customary to send the patient to a hospital or physician's office on those rare occasions when dental radiographs were prescribed. Not until 1914 did dental radiography become an accepted part of dental school curricula.

This limited use of dental radiography can be attributed both to the fact that the early equipment was primitive and sometimes dangerous, and to its widespread use as a means of entertainment by charlatans at fairgrounds. People often associated it with quackery. Resistance to change, ignorance, apathy, and fear delayed the widespread acceptance of radiography for years.

equipment improvements and new techniques

The quality of all x-ray units has improved steadily throughout the years. The newer units are more powerful than the old ones and produce better radiographs. Among recent developments are panoramic units, which are capable of exposing a radiograph of the entire dentition on a single film, and units whose tube heads are operated by remote controls. Improved film emulsions and processing chemicals have also enabled the radiographer to secure better radiographs and, at the same time, to shorten the exposure time. The recently introduced automatic dry film processor, which completely processes radiographs in four minutes or less, is gaining rapid acceptance.

Many innovations in dental radiography have improved techniques over the years. Two of the major problems that have plagued the dental radiographer were obtaining radiographs in which the teeth and related structures were shown in true anatomical relationship and size with minimal distortion, and prevention of the radiation beam from spreading to areas the dentist did not want to study. Both these problems now appear to be partly solved.

The first breakthrough took place in 1920 when Franklin McCormack developed the right angle, or paralleling, technique that greatly reduced dimensional distortion. Many others, notably Dr. G. M. Fitzgerald and Dr. William J. Updegrave, refined this technique and made it more practical. Dr. Updegrave has designed a series of film-positioning devices and written several booklets describing methods of simplifying the exposure of dental radiographs. Within the last few years major progress has been made in restricting the size of the x-ray beam. One such development is the replacing of the pointed cone through which x-rays pass from the tube head toward the patient with open circular lead-lined cones; another has been the introduction of rectangular lead-lined position indicating devices (PID) limiting the size of the x-ray beam that strikes the patient to the actual size of the dental film. Such a PID is shown in Fig. 1–1. Naturally, such devices are only effective if properly used and if all film exposure times and other factors that control radiation intensity are held to minimum required levels.

modern use of dental radiography

Few offices today are without x-ray units; many even have a unit in each operatory. The routine use of radiography enables the dentist to practice better dentistry. This obviously benefits the patient but also protects the dentist in the event of a dispute with the patient.

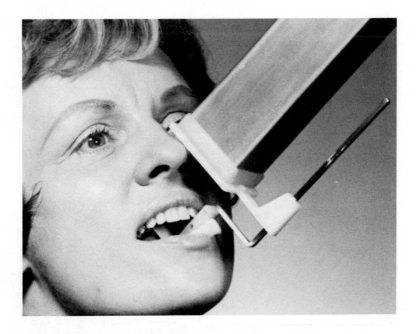

Fig. 1-1 Improved rectangular instrumentation for reduced tissue exposure. The radiographer first places the x-ray film on a holder, positions it in the oral cavity, and then brings the position indicating device (PID) into alignment with the indicator on the film holder by matching the slots and studs. The lead-lined PID limits the size of the x-ray beam to an area just large enough to exposure the film. (Courtesy of Rinn Corporation, Dental X-Ray Division.)

Radiographs are visible evidence of prior conditions or the nature of work performed and can be used as legal evidence. For this reason it is usually not good policy to give radiographs to a patient. Instead, when requested by the patient, such radiographs should be mailed to another dentist. The courts have ruled that radiographs are the property of the dentist; the patient pays only for the diagnosis. A related legal question is the frequency and number of radiographs that may be exposed. There is no set rule on this; the health and the needs of the patient are the determining factors.

It is difficult to imagine how any modern dental practice could be carried on without radiography (Fig. 1-2). At the same time no diagnosis can be based only on radiographic evidence. A visual and digital examination must always be made as well. But aside from helping the dental general practitioner make his diagnosis, radiographs help the prosthodontists and orthodontists to measure the head and to determine space relationships of the face. This type of radiograph is called a cephalometric headplate (from the Greek words *kephalē*, meaning

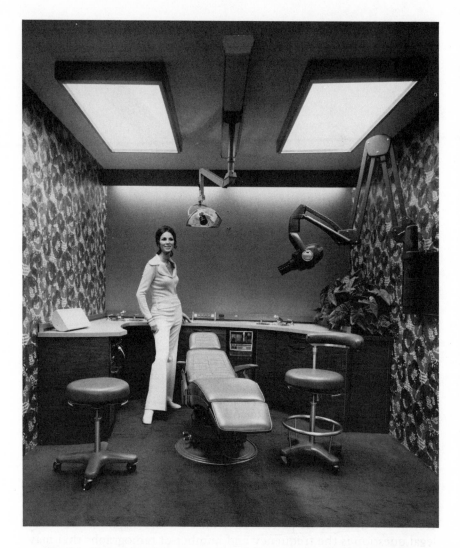

Fig. 1-2 Modern dental operatory with wall mounted x-ray machine. (Courtesy of Ritter Dental Manufacturing Company.)

"head," and *metricus*, meaning "measurement"). The oral surgeon depends on radiographs to locate fractures, impactions, foreign objects, and benign and malignant tumors. Every dental specialist makes use of radiographs at some time. The discovery of x-radiation has already revolutionized the practice of dentistry, and future technological advances undoubtedly will increase the use of radiography in the years ahead and make it safer.

bibliography

McCall, John Oppie, and Wald, Samuel Stanley. *Clinical Dental Roentgenology*, 4th ed. Philadelphia: W. P. Saunders Co., 1957.

Richardson, Richard E., and Barton, Roger E. *The Dental Assistant*, 4th ed. New York: McGraw-Hill Book Co., 1970.

Wainwright, William Ward. *Dental Radiology*, New York: McGraw-Hill Book Co., 1965.

Wuehrmann, Arthur H., and Manson-Hing, Lincoln R. *Dental Radiology*, 2d ed. St. Louis: The C. V. Mosby Co., 1969.

2

characteristics
of radiation

the physics of radiation

The scientist conceives the world to consist of matter and energy. Matter is defined as anything that occupies space and has mass. Thus all things that we see and recognize are forms of matter. Energy is defined as the ability to do work and overcome resistance. Heat, light, electricity, and x-radiation are forms of energy. Matter and energy are closely related. Energy is produced whenever the state of matter is altered by either natural or artificial means. The difference between water, steam, or ice is the amount of energy associated with the molecules. Such an energy exchange is produced within the x-ray machine and will be discussed later.

To understand radiation we must understand atomic structure. Currently we know of 104 basic elements occurring either singly or in combination in natural forms. Typical elements of interest in radiography are aluminum, copper, hydrogen, lead, oxygen, radium, and tungsten. Each of these elements is made up of atoms. An atom is the smallest particle of an element that still retains the properties of the element. If any given atom is split, the resulting components no longer retain the properties of the element. Atoms generally are combined with other atoms to form molecules. A molecule is the smallest particle of a substance that retains the properties of that substance. A simple molecule such as sodium chloride (table salt) contains only two atoms while a complex molecule may contain hundreds of atoms.

Atoms are extremely minute and are made up of a number of sub-atomic particles. For our purpose we are concerned only with the electrons, protons, and neutrons. *Electrons* have little mass or weight, are electrically negatively charged, and are constantly in motion. *Protons* weigh about 2,000 times as much as electrons and are electrically positively charged. *Neutrons* are a combination of one proton and one electron and are not electrically charged but neutral.

The atom's arrangement in some ways resembles the solar system. The atom has a nucleus as its center or sun and the electrons revolve around it like planets. The *nucleus* of all atoms except hydrogen contains at least one proton and one neutron (hydrogen in its simplest form has only a proton). Some atoms contain a very high number of each. The electrons and the nucleus normally remain in the same relative position to each other. To accommodate the electrons revolving about the nucleus, the larger atoms have several concentric orbits at various distances from the nucleus. These are referred to as "electron shells" which some chemists now call "energy levels." (The number of electrons in each of these spherical layers of energy varies, but is generally 2 in the first shell, 8 in the second, 18 in the third, 32 in the fourth, 50 in the fifth, and so on.) The innermost level is referred to as the K shell, the next as the L shell and so on. Only the K and L shells are important in dental radiography (Fig. 2-1). Their function will be explained later. Unless disturbed, as occurs

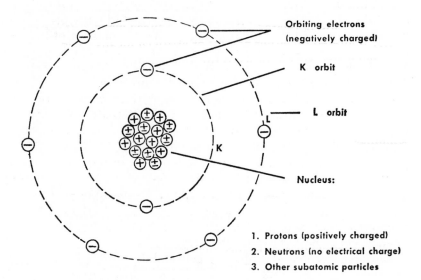

Fig. 2-1 Diagrammatic representation of an oxygen atom according to present fundamental concepts of matter. In the neutral atom, the number of positively-charged protons in the nucleus is equal to the number of negatively-charged orbiting electrons. (From Wuehrmann, Arthur H., and Manson-Hing, Lincoln R. *Dental Radiography*, 2d ed. St. Louis: The C. V. Mosby Co., 1969.)

when x-rays are produced, the electrons remain in their respective shells. The strong nuclear forces and magnetic attractions (binding energy) that attempt to draw them toward the nucleus are counterbalanced by the centrifugal forces caused by the revolving motion that attempt to pull them apart.

background and man-made radiation

Radiation is briefly defined as the process by which energy in the form of heat, light, electricity, or rays is sent out of atoms and molecules as they undergo internal change. This energy is emitted and propelled outwardly from its source in all directions (unless the direction is controlled as in the x-ray machine). This may occur spontaneously as with unstable elements such as radium or uranium or under man-made conditions.

A natural background radiation is present in our environment. We receive daily exposures of radiation from outer space in the form of light and many of the earth's materials are radioactive. To understand radioactivity we must realize that while most elements are stable, a few undergo constant spontaneous changes. As we have already seen, each atom of a certain element has an equal number of protons and electrons. Tungsten, the metal most concerned in x-ray production, has 74 protons and 74 electrons and a constant number of neutrons. However, variations occur in some elements. For example, the majority of hydrogen atoms contain no neutrons but two rarer forms exist. The first of these, deuterium, contains a neutron in its nucleus and is stable. The second and much rarer form, tritium, contains two neutrons and is unstable and radioactive. Such alternate forms are called *isotopes.* Each isotope of a specific atom has the same chemical properties: they differ only in mass and weight (Fig. 2-2).

Most elements are now believed to have one or more isotopes: over 1,500 of these have already been identified. Of these, over half are unstable and radioactive. Instability in an atom can be natural or man-made; either type is important to medicine and dentistry. Many dental schools are conducting research with radioactive isotopes and much is yet to be discovered about them.

Unstable isotopes attempt to regain stability through the release of energy, by a process known as decay in which the unstable nucleus of the isotope continues to decay (give off radiation) until stability of the nucleus is attained. This decay process involves the giving off of two distinct forms of radiation: particulate radiation consisting of bits of matter traveling at high speeds (also called corpuscular radia-

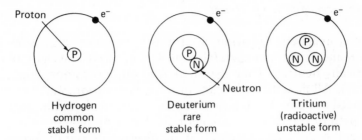

Fig. 2-2 Isotopes of hydrogen. Approximately 1 in 14,000 hydrogen atoms contain 1 neutron in the nucleus (deuterium). Another rare hydrogen atom is tritium, which contains 2 neutrons in the nucleus. Each of these isotopes has the same chemical properties, but they differ in physical mass and weight. Unstable isotopes seek to become stable by a release of energy through a process known as decay. This process involves giving off two kinds of radiation: corpuscular or particulate radiation and electromagnetic radiation.

tion), and electromagnetic radiation which is a combination of electric and magnetic energy and is emitted in the form of rays or waves.

Particulate radiation originates from naturally occurring isotopes and is given off in the form of alpha particles, beta particles, and neutrons. The alpha particles which contain two protons and two neutrons are positively charged and are much heavier than the beta particles which are high speed negatively charged electrons. As already indicated, neutrons are uncharged.

Another form of naturally occurring radiation belongs to the family of electromagnetic radiation and is called *gamma radiation.* Gamma rays are very similar to x-rays but occur naturally while x-rays are man-made. Gamma rays normally possess greater energy and penetrating power than x-rays. A further difference is that gamma rays originate from the nucleus whereas x-rays originate from electrons. Although radioactive isotopes are frequently used in hospitals and are also being used by dentists in some research and teaching centers, our concern is with the man-made forms of radiation; the information on natural radiation is included for the sake of completeness in presenting a proper background to the study of radiography.

Man has learned to produce several types of radiations which are identical to natural radiations. Although our main concern deals with x-radiation, ultraviolet waves are also produced artificially for sun lamps or fluorescent lights, and for numerous other uses. One of the most recent man-made radiations is the laser beam whose potential is not fully known at this time. We can confidently await the development of further man-made radiations.

the electromagnetic spectrum

Electromagnetic radiations are forms of radiant energy, some natural and some man-made, that possess no mass or weight and are electrically neutral. They also share four other common characteristics: 1. All pass through space in wave-like motion; 2. All travel at the speed of light; 3. All give off an electrical field at right angles to their path of travel, and a magnetic field at right angles to the electric field; 4. All have energies that are measurable and different.

The basic differences between types of electromagnetic radiation are their wavelengths and frequencies. One determines wavelengths by measuring the distance from the crest of one wave to the crest of the following one, and frequency by measuring the number of oscillations per second (Fig. 2-3). Each form of electromagnetic radiation has its own wavelength and frequency which indicate its main property, source, or use. When wavelength and frequency change, the characteristics of the radiation also change.

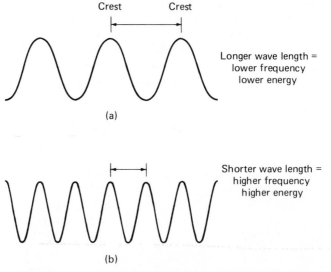

Fig. 2-3 Differences in wavelengths and frequencies. Only the shortest wavelengths with extremely high frequency and energy are used to expose film in dental radiography. Wavelength is determined by the distances between the crests. Observe that this distance is much shorter in B than in A. The photons that comprise the dental x-ray beam are estimated to have over 250 million such crests per inch. (From Kinsman, Simon, and Alcox, Ray W. *Radiation Hygiene in Dental Practice.* Sacramento: State of California, Department of Public Health, Bureau of Radiological Health, 1970.)

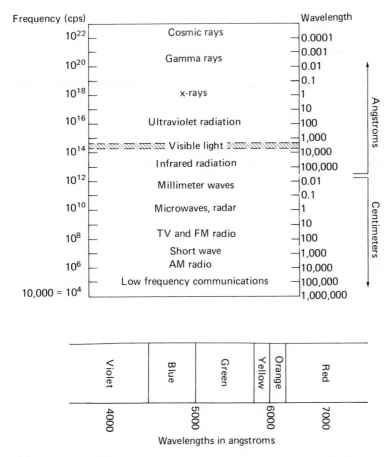

Fig. 2-4 The electromagnetic spectrum. (From Kinsman, Simon, and Alcox, Ray W. *Radiation Hygiene in Dental Practice*. Sacramento: State of California, Department of Public Health, Bureau of Radiological Health, 1970.)

The electromagnetic spectrum consists of an orderly arrangement of all known radiant energies (Fig. 2-4). For convenience these are portrayed according to their wavelengths. The longest wavelengths, which are those used for low frequency communications, are so long that they are best measured in kilometers (each kilometer is a thousand meters or about 5/8 mile), while the shortest cosmic rays are measured in Angstrom units (one Å is about 1/250,000,000 inch or 1/100,000,000 centimeter). No clear-cut separation exists between the various radiations represented on the electromagnetic spectrum; consequently overlapping of the wavelengths is common. Each form of radiation has a range of frequencies; that accounts for some of the longer infrared waves being measured in meters while the shorter infrared waves are measured in Angstrom units. It therefore follows that all x-radiations are not the same length. The longest of these are the Grenz rays, also called soft radiation, that have only limited penetrating power and are unsuitable for exposing dental radiographs. The wavelengths used in diagnostic dental radiography range from about 0.1 to 0.5 Å and are classified as hard radiation, a term meaning radiation with great penetrating power. Even still shorter wavelengths are produced by supervoltage machines used when still greater penetration is required as in some forms of medical therapy and industrial radiography.

characteristics of x-radiation

X-rays are believed to consist of minute bundles of pure energy called *photons* (or quanta). These have no mass or weight, are invisible, and cannot be sensed. Because they travel at the speed of light (186,000 miles per second), these x-ray photons are often referred to as "bullets of energy."

Bodies in motion are believed to have *kinetic* energy (from the Greek *kineticos*, "pertaining to motion"). As already discussed, the electrons of any atom are in continuous motion within their orbital shells or energy levels around the nucleus. The velocity of this motion is drastically increased as the temperature is raised; this happens within the x-ray tube when its components are heated by a high-voltage current and free electrons are propelled at extremely high speeds toward a tungsten target. The particular area of the target toward which these electrons are directed is the focal spot; it is here that the x-ray originates. The details of the x-ray tube, focal spot, and the methods by which the electrons cross the tube will be explained in detail in Chapters 3 and 4.

A form of energy transfer takes place within the x-ray tube as the electrons are either stopped or slowed down by impact with the tungsten target in which all or part of the kinetic energy is given up. However, since energy is always present in nature and can actually never be created or destroyed, the so-called "lost" kinetic energy is actually converted at the focal spot into heat and x-rays. Unfortunately, less than 1 percent of this converted energy is released in the form of useful x-ray photons; the other 99 percent is in useless heat.

The amount and type of energy released during energy conversion depend upon the manner in which the electrons strike the atoms of the target. At any given moment a slight difference in potential (the

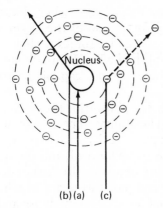

Fig. 2-5 Electrons colliding with simulated tungsten atom (number of electrons is insufficient for this atom to be tungsten). (a) Giving up all of its energy; (b) relinquishing part of its energy; (c) displacing a K shell (orbit) electron. (From Wuehrmann, Arthur H., and Manson-Hing, Lincoln R. *Dental Radiology*, 2d ed. St. Louis: The C. V. Mosby Co., 1969.)

(b)(a)   (c)

strength of the current) may alter the speed at which the free electrons are accelerated across the tube. All electrons hitting the target are not decelerated in the same degree. Some are absorbed by the target atoms, some are slowed down, and others are deviated from their path of travel (Fig. 2-5). Thus the x-ray beam formed at the focal spot is polychromatic; that is, it contains x-ray photons of various energies and penetrating power.

The degree of acceleration, the manner of impact at the focal spot, and the binding energy determine the type of wavelength that is produced. The term *binding* energy is used to describe the force which maintains the electrons in their relative positions around the nucleus. This binding energy increases the closer the electron is to the nucleus. An electron from the inner K shell is more tightly held in position near the nucleus than an electron from the L shell or another of the outer shells; therefore it takes more energy to remove a K electron. The binding energy is not always the same from atom to atom and the electrons of each shell have slightly different kinetic characteristics. In the event that the manner of impact forces a K electron into space, it is replaced by an electron from the L shell.

The conversion of kinetic energy into x-ray photons is accomplished in two ways within the dental x-ray tube. The first and most important for dental radiography is called *Bremsstrahlung* (German for braking radiation). When a free electron collides with the nucleus of an atom in the target metal and cannot travel further, it gives up all of its energy in the form of very short wavelengths—the most powerful type produced by the dental x-ray machine. However, if the electron has a glancing collision with the target atom and gives up only part of its kinetic energy, the x-rays produced will have longer wavelengths, less energy and penetrating power. The majority of x-rays produced by dental machines are formed by these types of collisions. The second way, *characteristic radiation,* is when the free electron collides with an orbiting K electron instead of the target atom and the electron from the L shell replaces it and assumes K shell characteristics. This can only be accomplished when high-voltage currents are used. All dental x-ray machines are not capable of utilizing such voltages.

Another important characteristic of x-ray photons is the ability to pass through gases, liquids, and solids. The ability to penetrate materials or tissues depends on the wavelength, the distance between the source of the x-ray and the object that is to be x-rayed, and the density of the object. The composition of the object or the tissues determines whether the x-rays will penetrate and pass through it or whether they will be absorbed in it. Materials that are extremely dense and have a high atomic number will absorb more x-rays than thin materials with low atomic numbers. This partially explains why dense structures such as bone and enamel appear radiopaque (white or light) on the radiograph, whereas the less dense pulp chamber, muscles, and skin appear radiolucent (dark or black). Some of the x-ray photons interact with the materials that they penetrate. This interaction is called ionization or the formation of ions.

ionizing radiation

Ions are defined as electrically charged atoms or electrons. The formation of ions is easier to understand if we first review the normal structural arrangement of the atom. The atom normally has the same number of protons (positive charges) in the nucleus as it has electrons (negative charges) in the orbital shells. If one of these electrons is separated from its orbit around the nucleus, the remainder of the atom loses its electrical neutrality. An atom from which an electron has been removed has more protons than electrons, is positively charged, and is called a positive ion. The negatively charged electron that has been separated from the atom is called a negative ion. Together they are called an ion pair. When an atom is struck by an x-ray photon, an electron may be dislodged and an ion pair created (Fig. 2-6). As high energy electrons travel on, electrons from other atoms may be ejected in a chain reaction creating additional ion pairs. These unstable ions attempt to regain electrical stability by combining with another oppositely charged ion with the result that new atomic combinations are occasionally created.

Any radiation that produces ions is called *radiation ionization.* Only a portion of the radiations portrayed on the electromagnetic spectrum, the x-rays, alpha and beta particles, and the gamma and

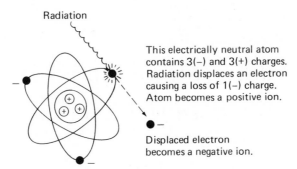

Radiation

This electrically neutral atom contains 3(–) and 3(+) charges. Radiation displaces an electron causing a loss of 1(–) charge. Atom becomes a positive ion.

Displaced electron becomes a negative ion.

Fig. 2-6 Ionization, showing the removal of an orbital electron by the kinetic energy of radiation. (From Kinsman, Simon, and Alcox, Ray W. *Radiation Hygiene in Dental Practice*. Sacramento: State of California, Department of Public Health, Bureau of Radiological Health, 1970.)

cosmic rays, are of the ionizing type. In dental radiography our concern is limited to the possible changes that may occur in the cellular structures of the tissues as ions are produced through the passage of x-rays through the cells. Occasionally these ions recombine to form new tissues; the mechanics of biological tissue damage will be further explained in Chapter 5.

bibliography

Ennis, Leroy M., Berry, Harrison M., and Phillips, James E. *Dental Roentgenology*, 6th ed. Philadelphia: Lea & Febiger, 1967.

Kinsman, Simon, and Alcox, Ray W. *Radiation Hygiene in Dental Radiography*, Sacramento: State of California, Department of Public Health, Bureau of Radiological Health, 1970.

O'Brien, Richard C. *Dental Radiography*, 2d ed. Philadelphia: W. B. Saunders Co., 1972.

Peterson, Shailer. *Clinical Dental Hygiene,* 3d ed. St. Louis: The C. V. Mosby Co., 1968.

Wainwright, William Ward. *Dental Radiology,* 2d ed. New York: McGraw-Hill Book Co., 1965.

Wuehrmann, Arthur H., and Manson-Hing, Lincoln R. *Dental Radiology*, 2d ed. St. Louis: The C. V. Mosby Co., 1969.

3

the dental x-ray machine–
components and functions

The x-ray machine has gone through a long period of development. The unreliable gas tubes used in the older machines gave way to the vastly improved Coolidge tube, a thermionic emission (the creation of ions by heat) tube invented by Dr. W. D. Coolidge, and the old machines with exposed high tension wires are now museum relics. Much scientific study and extensive research have resulted in a modern dental x-ray machine that is safe, compact, effective, easy to position, and easy to operate. To understand how x-rays are produced, one must understand the components of the dental x-ray machine and its functions.

Many manufacturers, domestic and foreign, offer a variety of x-ray machine models and accessories. All x-ray machines—whether mobile or stationary—whether mounted on the wall, the floor, or the ceiling—operate on similar principles. The greatest differences between them are their size, their voltage range, and their regulating controls.

The x-ray machines used in hospitals and industry are often much larger than those used in dental offices. The variations in size and electric potential (voltage) are dictated by the amount of penetration of tissue that is required. The low-voltage machines, with a voltage range from 10,000 to 20,000 volts, are used to radiograph substances with rather low density. The higher-voltage machines, with a voltage range from 45,000 to 100,000 volts, are used in dentistry for better tissue penetration. Supervoltage machines, with ranges up to 3 million volts, are used in hospitals and in industry.

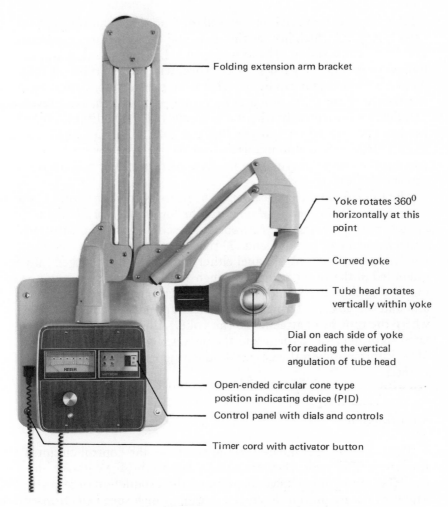

Folding extension arm bracket

Yoke rotates 360^0 horizontally at this point

Curved yoke

Tube head rotates vertically within yoke

Dial on each side of yoke for reading the vertical angulation of tube head

Open-ended circular cone type position indicating device (PID)

Control panel with dials and controls

Timer cord with activator button

Fig. 3-1 Typical wall mounted dental x-ray machine. (Courtesy of Ritter Dental Manufacturing Company.)

parts and components

Most dental x-ray machines are similar in size and appearance and have similar structural components and electrical parts (Fig. 3-1). All these parts may vary in size, shape, and arrangement. The standard structural parts include (1) a *control panel* which may be a

cabinet, a panel mounted on the wall, or a portable control box,
(2) a *tube head* which houses the tube, and (3) a flexible *extension
arm* from which the tube head is suspended. The extension arm is
hollow to permit the passage of electrical wires to the tube. It folds
up like a bracket and can be swiveled from side to side. The tube head
is attached to the extension arm by means of a yoke that can revolve
360 degrees horizontally where it is connected. In addition, the tube
head can be rotated vertically within the yoke. The tube head is made
of cast metal (often aluminum) and protectively lined with lead to
prevent the escape of radiation in any direction except toward the
position indicating device.

The fundamental electrical parts of the x-ray machine are: (1) the
x-ray tube, (2) the *electrical circuits* (the low-voltage or filament
circuit, the high-voltage or cathode-anode circuit, and the autotransformer or control circuit), and (3) the *timing device*. The electric
current enters the control panel either through a cord plugged into a
grounded outlet in the wall or through a direct connection to a power
line in the wall. It continues to and through the hollow extension
arm and the *yoke*, entering the tube head from both sides at a point
where the tube head attaches to the yoke. All areas are heavily insulated to protect the patient and the operator from electrical shock.
More information on the circuits and wiring is provided later in this
chapter.

the x-ray tube

The tube can be compared to the heart and the control circuits to
the arteries and veins; they are equally important, for without one
the other could not achieve its purpose, the production of x-rays.
These x-rays are produced when a stream of high speed electrons strikes
a target. Four conditions must exist for x-rays to be produced: (1) a
source of free electrons, (2) high-voltage to impart speed to them,
(3) a concentration of electrons into a small area, and (4) a target
that is capable of stopping them. The x-ray tube and the circuits
within the machine are designed to create these conditions.

The earliest tubes used in radiography were glass bulbs from which
the air had been only partially evacuated and replaced with hydrogen
or some other gas. An *anode* (the positive terminal or electrode in an
electric circuit) and a *cathode* (the negative terminal or electrode)
were sealed within the tube and the two protruding arms of the elec-

trodes permitted the passage of the current through the tube. The electron supply was dependent upon the ionization of gases within the tube when it was in operation. The current flowing between these *electrodes* from cathode to anode was called the *cathode stream*. Because the air evacuation was only partial, these early tubes were quite erratic in their operation, working well one day and not at all the next. A major breakthrough was the invention in 1913 of the Coolidge tube, an improved model which is still in use in most of today's x-ray machines.

The design of the Coolidge tube eliminated the need for gas to create electrons, replacing gas with an incandescent (glowing with heat) filament in the cathode. This process, known as *thermionic emission,* occurs whenever a wire is heated to incandescence. Literally boiled out of the wire, the electrodes form a cloud around it. A familiar example of this phenomenon is the tungsten electric light bulb we all use. The operator can accurately control the thermionic emission produced in the improved, highly evacuated Coolidge tube by determining how hot the filament in the cathode should be.

The x-ray tube, located inside the tube head, is a glass bulb from which the air has been pumped out to create a vacuum. The vacuum offers a minimum resistance to the stream of electrons flowing across the space between the two electrodes sealed in the tube and facing each other. In most x-ray machines used in the United States the space between the electrons is less than one inch. The cathode and the anode are connected to the outside of the tube by massive copper wires, which permit a high-voltage current to flow across the tube when the x-ray machine is in operation (Fig. 3–2).

A metal housing surrounds the x-ray tube and performs several important functions: (1) it protects the tube from accidental damage, (2) it increases the safety of the x-ray machine by grounding its high-voltage components (the x-ray tube and the transformers) to prevent shock, (3) it prevents overheating and prolongs the useful life of the x-ray tube by providing a space filled with oil or air to absorb the heat that is produced during the energy conversion in which the electrons give off x-rays and heat (some x-ray machines are air-cooled), and (4) it reduces to an acceptable level the amount of primary radiation which is produced during the operation of the tube and which is permitted to exit from it.

The cathode assembly at the negative end of the tube consists of a thin spiral filament of tungsten wire about 1/2 inch long. This filament, when heated to incandescence, produces the electrons. The

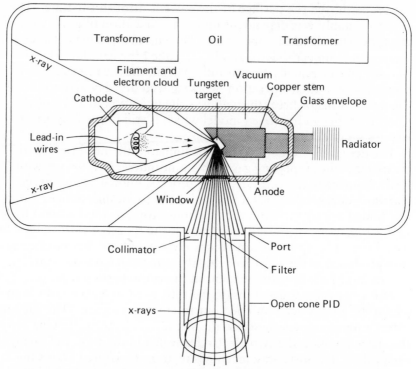

Fig. 3–2 Representation of a dental x-ray tube housing, dental x-ray tube, electron beam, and x-ray beam. When an electric current is applied to the high-voltage circuit (between the anode and the cathode), each electron is propelled from the cathode to the target on the anode, producing heat and x-rays. (From Kinsman, Simon, and Alcox, Ray W. *Radiation Hygiene in Dental Practice.* Sacramento: State of California, Department of Public Health, Bureau of Radiological Health, 1970.)

wire filament is recessed into a molybdenum *focusing cup,* which directs the electrons toward the target on the anode (Fig. 3–3).

The anode assembly on the positive end of the tube consists of a copper bar with a tungsten button imbedded in the end that faces the focusing cup of the cathode. On dental x-ray machines this tungsten button, called the *target*, is set into the copper at an angle of 20 degrees to the cathode. Various other target angles are used for industrial or special purpose x-ray machines.

Of major importance to the dental radiographer is a small area on the *target* that the electrons strike to produce x-rays. When the tube is in operation, a cloud of electrons first forms around the filament wire of the cathode as the tube warms. Later, when the high-voltage current is applied, these electrons are attracted and propelled toward a rectangular area on the surface of the target. This area is known as

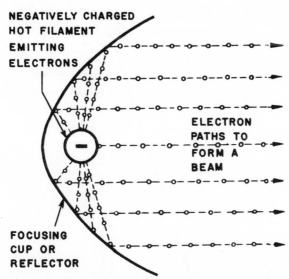

NEGATIVELY CHARGED HOT FILAMENT EMITTING ELECTRONS

ELECTRON PATHS TO FORM A BEAM

FOCUSING CUP OR REFLECTOR

Fig. 3-3 Formation of electron beam by focusing device. The filament is placed in a reflector or focusing cup within the cathode structure, which focuses the electron beam in a similar manner to light focused by a flashlight reflector. When the high-voltage circuit is activated, an electromotive or potential difference between the cathode and the anode is established and the free electrons are accelerated toward the focal spot on the anode target at approximately 1/2 the speed of light. (Courtesy of General Electric, Medical Systems Division.)

the *focal spot*. Its size can be controlled by the manufacturer, who determines the shape and size of the tungsten filament wire and the angle at which the target faces it. A small focal spot not only improves the definition (sharpness) on the radiograph but also concentrates the electrons and permits the use of higher voltage with less damage to the tube. The size of the focal spot is effectively reduced by the application of the line-focus principle (Fig. 3–4). This involves focusing the electron stream and directing it into the narrow rectangle on the face of the target on the anode. If one were to stand directly beneath the x-ray tube and look up at it, the rectangular focal spot would appear square. The purpose of the line-focus is to generate x-rays over a large area for better heat dissipation.

principles of x-ray tube operation

A low-voltage current passes through the filament circuit of the x-ray tube as soon as the machine is turned on. This causes the tungsten filament in the focusing cup of the cathode to glow with heat and form the electron cloud. Thus the filament is already hot and

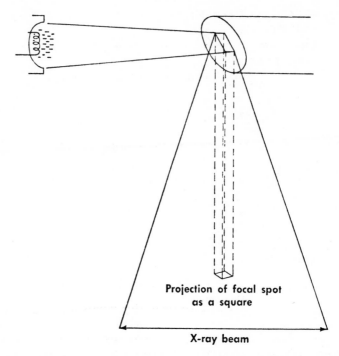

Projection of focal spot
as a square

X-ray beam

Fig. 3–4 Representation of the anode, focal spot, and x-ray beams. As seen from points within the x-ray beam, the focal spot appears as a square of approximately 0.8 × 0.8 mm. This square is the source of radiation or effective focal spot for the beam of radiation. The actual focal spot is rectangular and has a considerably greater area (approximately 0.8 × 0.18 mm). (From Wuehrmann, Arthur H., and Manson-Hing, Lincoln R. *Dental Radiography*, 2d ed. St. Louis: The C. V. Mosby Co., 1969.)

"boiling off" electrons before the x-ray machine is activated to produce x-rays. This phase of the operation in which the electron cloud of free electrons forms can be compared to warming up the engine on a car. By depressing the activator button on the end of the timer cord the second and final phase of the operation that results in the production of x-rays is begun; this corresponds to stepping on the accelerator on the car and getting into motion. As high voltage (a difference in electrical pressure) is applied to the space between the two electrodes (cathode and anode) the free electrons which are negative are attracted to the positive anode and travel across the space to the anode at approximately half the speed of light. As we have already seen, the focusing cup in the cathode focuses the electrons onto the small focal spot on the target. These high-velocity electrons disturb the tungsten atoms in the target and this energy is converted into 99 percent heat and 1 percent x-rays. The metal tungsten (symbol W and atomic weight 74—also known as Wolfram) is ideally suited for use in the filament and target because it can withstand extremely high temperatures (melting point 3370 degrees Celsius). Its high atomic number makes it possible to liberate electrons easily from their orbital shells when the metal is heated. Because tungsten is a poor conductor of heat, the tungsten button is always imbedded in a stem or core of copper. Copper is highly conductive and carries the heat off to the *radiator* which is just outside the tube (refer to the tube diagram). In an oil-cooled tube the large mass of copper in which the tungsten is imbedded conducts the heat out of the tube into a radiator that transfers the heat to the oil surrounding the tube; in an air-cooled tube the heat is transferred through the copper and the radiator into the air inside the tube head.

The x-rays produced by the energy exchange within the tube are emitted in all directions within the tube head. Many of these rays bounce around inside the tube head until they are absorbed by the oil, air, wires, transformers, or the tube head lining. A window (a thin area in the glass envelope) is located at a point where the emission of x-rays is most intense. In turn, this window is aligned with an opening in the tube head called the *aperture* or *port* that is covered by a permanent seal of glass, beryllium, or aluminum. If the tube head is properly sealed, the aperture is the only place through which the x-rays can escape the tube head. The PID fits over the aperture and can be moved to aim the central beam of radiation in the desired direction.

voltage

Voltage is the electrical pressure or potential difference between two electrical charges. In radiography this difference in potential determines the electromotive force (the force which attracts the electrons to the anode) and the speed of the electrons when traveling from cathode to anode. This speed of the electrons, in turn, determines the energy (penetrating power) of the x-rays produced. When the voltage is increased, the electrons travel faster and produce the hardest type radiation.

The *volt* is the unit of electromotive force used to measure the electrical potential. It is defined as the electromotive force sufficient to cause one ampere of current to flow against a resistance of one ohm (the ampere is a measure of amount of current; the ohm is a measure of resistance). Because dental x-ray equipment operates at very high voltages, it is customary to express voltage in terms of *kilovolts*. The kilovolt equals 1,000 volts and is abbreviated *kV*. The voltage varies during an exposure producing a polychromatic beam containing high energy rays and also containing some rays that have barely enough energy to escape from the tube. The highest voltage to which the current in the tube rises during an exposure is called the kilovolt peak, abbreviated *kVp.* Thus if the x-ray machine controls are set at 65,000 volts, the maximum x-ray energy that can be produced during this exposure is 65 kVp.

amperage

The ampere is the unit of quantity of electric current. An increase in amperage results in an increase in the number of electrons that are available to travel from the cathode to anode when the tube is activated, and this results in a production of more x-rays. Only a small current is required to operate the x-ray machine; therefore, the term *milliampere* denoting 1/1000 of an ampere is used. This is abbreviated *mA.* The majority of dental x-ray machines operate at 10 or 15 mA. The milliamperage can be adjusted on most x-ray machines.

electric current

Electric current can flow in either direction along a wire or conductor; it can flow steadily in one direction or flow in pulses and change directions. *Direct current,* abbreviated *DC,* flows continuously in one direction. Such a unidirectional current is used in flashlight batteries for example, but cannot be used in the dental x-ray machine unless modifications are made to the machine.

The ordinary household current used in most parts of the United States is a 110 volt and 60 cycle *alternating current,* abbreviated *AC,* that changes its direction of flow 60 times per second; thus the alternating current has two phases—one positive and the other negative—and alternates between these phases. With the exception of x-ray machines modified or designed for use in remote places or military field hospitals, most dental x-ray machines operate on alternating current. Although it is customary to describe the cathode as the negative electrode and the anode as the positive electrode, this is not quite the case during the time that the x-ray tube is producing x-rays because the cathode and the anode each change from negative to positive 60 times per second. Since free electrons are available only at the cathode filament, x-rays can be produced only when the electrons flow across the gap from cathode to anode during the phase when the anode is positive. Theoretically, when the cycle reverses any available electrons would flow back to the cathode; however, x-rays cannot be produced when the anode is in the negative phase because no free electrons are available at the target on the anode to be carried back across the gap to the cathode, and the current is thus blocked from traveling in that direction.

Actually this alternation in current direction which occurs every 1/120 second (twice during each full cycle) is very beneficial because it produces the x-rays in a series of bursts or pulses rather than in a continuous flow which would overheat and damage the tube. The term *rectification* is used to describe the process in which the current is unidirectional. Because no special rectifying tubes or devices are used, x-ray equipment which operates only to produce x-rays during half of each cycle is known as "self rectifying" (Fig. 3–5).

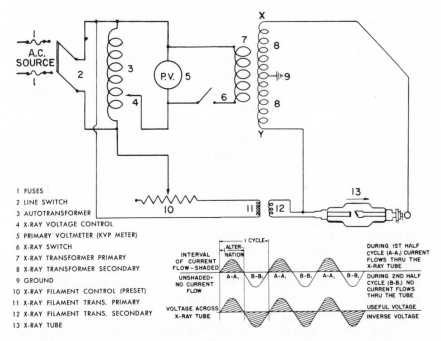

1 FUSES
2 LINE SWITCH
3 AUTOTRANSFORMER
4 X-RAY VOLTAGE CONTROL
5 PRIMARY VOLTMETER (KVP METER)
6 X-RAY SWITCH
7 X-RAY TRANSFORMER PRIMARY
8 X-RAY TRANSFORMER SECONDARY
9 GROUND
10 X-RAY FILAMENT CONTROL (PRESET)
11 X-RAY FILAMENT TRANS. PRIMARY
12 X-RAY FILAMENT TRANS. SECONDARY
13 X-RAY TUBE

Fig. 3–5 The basic x-ray unit consisting of three types of transformers, the x-ray tube, and several additional devices. For explanatory purposes, the basic circuit is divided into the filament (low-voltage) circuit, the anode-cathode (high-voltage) circuit, and the timing circuit. Ordinary household electric current is called 60 cycle alternating current because the current changes direction of flow 60 times a second. Alternating current can be shown in wave form. The crest of the wave represents the maximum voltage when the current is moving in one direction while the trough of the wave represents the maximum voltage when the current is moving in the other direction. The total cycle takes place in 1/60 of a second. (Courtesy of General Electric, Medical Systems Division.)

transformers

As already shown, each dental x-ray machine has a low-voltage filament circuit and a high-voltage cathode-anode circuit. A series of transformers are required to decrease (step-down) or increase (step-up) the ordinary 110-volt current that enters the x-ray machine. A *transformer* is an electromagnetic device for changing the alternating current and consists of two coils of electric wire wound on an iron core. The primary coil is connected to the alternating current supply, and the secondary coil is connected to the tube circuit. The wires in these coils are insulated from each other. When the current is flowing, a magnetic field from around the primary coil induces an electric current in the secondary coil. The secondary voltage thus created can be accurately predicted. The number of wire turns in each coil determines whether the voltage is decreased or increased. For example, if there are ten times more turns on the primary than on the secondary coil, the voltage is decreased tenfold; if the ratio is reversed, the voltage increases tenfold.

A low-voltage (step-down) transformer (shown as items 11 and 12 in Fig. 3–5) decreases the current to between 3 and 12 volts, depending on the make of the machine. A rheostat or choke coil (item 10 in Fig. 3–5) hinders the passage of electricity and reduces or controls the amount of current (amperage) flowing in the circuit. This low-voltage current begins to flow through the filament circuit when the line switch of the x-ray machine is turned on, and is sufficient to heat the cathode filament and form the electron cloud.

A high-voltage (step-up) transformer (items 7 and 8 in Fig. 3–5) increases the current as required by the technique the radiographer is using. Although the use of higher voltage has steadily increased, the majority of exposures are made with 65,000 volts. The high-voltage current begins to flow through the cathode-anode circuit when the activator button is depressed and is essential to propel the electrons toward the target.

An *autotransformer* is a voltage compensator that corrects minor fluctuations in the current flowing through the wires. Like the transformers, it has an iron core but is wound with only a single coil that does the work of two (item 3 in Fig. 3–5). The action of the autotransformer is based on *self-induction* in a single coil rather than on mutual induction produced between two coils with different numbers of turns. By turning a knob on the control panel, the operator causes a selector switch to slide over a series of tabs and regulates the voltage by either decreasing or increasing it. This action compares to fine tuning on a radio.

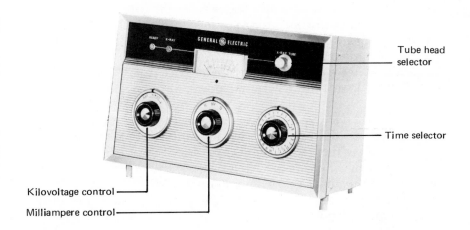

Tube head
selector

Time selector

Kilovoltage control

Milliampere control

Fig. 3–6 A typical modern x-ray control box that is movable and capable of operating x-ray machines in three separate locations. (Courtesy of General Electric, Medical Systems Division.)

control devices

The regulatory control devices vary greatly according to the manufacturer, some even offering a choice of differently designed and equipment control panels. However, there are four major controls that must be operated on most variable-type dental x-ray machines—the line switch to the electrical outlet, the milliammeter, the voltmeter, and a timer (Fig. 3–6).

The *line switch* is usually a toggle switch that can be flicked on or off with light finger pressure. It is generally located on the side or face of the cabinet or control panel. On most machines a small red light turns on to warn that the machine is operational. At the same time the needle on the voltmeter moves to indicate that current is reaching the machine.

The *milliammeter* or ammeter, as it is often called, measures the amount of current passing through the wires of the circuit. Mathematically, amperage is a linear factor expressed in the first power; that means, if amperage is doubled the radiation produced is also doubled. The milliampere selector can be adjusted to increase or decrease the milliamperage.

The *voltmeter* measures the electromotive force (the difference in potential or voltage across the x-ray tube; actually the difference between the primary and secondary coils in the high-voltage transformer).

A kilovolt peak selector, in the form of pushbuttons, knobs, or dials, controls the tabs that slide over the turns of the wire in the autotransformer and enable the operator to change the peak kilovoltage. Mathematically, voltage is an exponential factor. For example, doubling the kilovoltage would result in far more than twice as much penetrating power. For practical purposes, an increase from 70 to 80 kVp is sufficient to double the penetrating power of the x-rays that are produced.

The *timer* serves to regulate the duration of the interval that the current will pass through the x-ray tube, thus enabling the operator to predetermine the length of the exposure. The timer switches on dental x-ray machines are mechanical, electrical, or electronic. One sets most of them by turning a pointer on the dial or by turning the dial itself counterclockwise. Depending on the age and model of the x-ray machine, exposures from as low as 1/60 second to 5 seconds may be selected. The older mechanical timers, many of which are still in use, operate with a spring mechanism which is not consistently accurate at time intervals of less than a second. Some mechanical timers are reasonably accurate at intervals as low as 1/4 second. These are quite satisfactory when slow film is used; however, film manufacturers have constantly improved film quality and decreased the time required to expose films. With the use of extra-high speed films, exposure times as low as 1/20 second are common. These short intervals cannot be measured by mechanical timers and require either electrical or electronic timers. An activator button is located on the handle of the timer cord. All dental x-ray machines are required to be equipped with an exposure switch of the "deadman" type, which automatically terminates the exposure when the finger ceases to press on the timer button. This makes it necessary to maintain firm pressure on the button during the entire exposure. Failure to do so results in the formation of an insufficient number of x-rays to properly expose the film. Ideally, the timer cord should be sufficiently long to enable the operator to step into an area of radiation safety (normally at least six feet from the source of the x-ray beam). By observing the dial on the milliammeter indicator, it is possible to determine whether x-rays are being generated.

The present trend is toward simpler and automated controls. An example of this is the electrical timer which automatically resets itself and does not have to be altered unless a change in the exposure time is desired. This makes operation easier and results more consistent.

The operation of each x-ray machine is explained fully in the operating manual provided by the manufacturer. The operator should study it until he is thoroughly familiar with the operational capability and maintenance requirements of the machine.

bibliography

Ennis, Leroy M., Berry, Harrison M., and Phillips, James E. *Dental Roentgenology*, 6th ed. Philadelphia: Lea & Febiger, 1967.

Kinsman, Simon, and Alcox, Ray W. *Radiation Hygiene in Dental Radiography*, Sacramento: State of California, Department of Public Health, Bureau of Radiological Health, 1970.

Peterson, Shailer. *Clinical Dental Hygiene*, 3d ed. St. Louis: The C. V. Mosby Co., 1968.

Richardson, Richard E., and Barton, Roger E. *The Dental Assistant*, 4th ed. New York: McGraw-Hill Book Co., 1970.

Wilkins, Esther M. *Clinical Practice of the Dental Hygienist*, 3d ed. Philadelphia: Lea & Febiger, 1971.

Wuehrmann, Arthur H., and Manson-Hing, Lincoln R. *Dental Radiology*, 2d ed. St. Louis: The C. V. Mosby Co., 1969.

X-Ray Generation and Radiographic Principles in Dentistry, Milwaukee: General Electric Company, Technical Services, X-Ray Department.

X-Rays in Dentistry, Rochester, N.Y.: Eastman Kodak Co., 1972.

4

technical aspects
of radiation production

operation of the dental x-ray machine

A summation of the fundamentals of x-ray generation is in order before considering the technical aspects of radiation production. In review, when the line switch of the x-ray machine is turned on, the line current enters the filament circuit of the x-ray machine. A step-down transformer reduces the voltage before it enters the circuit and heats the filament of the cathode to incandescence, separating electrons from their atoms. The degree to which the filament is heated depends upon the milliamperage that is selected—the higher the mA, the more electrons in the electron cloud. These electrons are now in a state of excitation as they hover around the filament wire. X-rays are not produced until the activator button on the end of the timer cord is pressed. When this occurs, the line current enters the cathode-anode circuit. A step-up transformer then increases the voltage to impart sufficient force to propel the free electrons to the focal spot on the anode where the energy conversion takes place resulting in the production of x-rays and energy. The x-ray beam formed at the focal spot is polychromatic, consisting of wavelengths of various energies. The higher the voltage, the greater the penetration power of the x-rays that are formed.

To achieve consistent results, the x-ray machine operator should always follow an orderly procedure. These steps are listed here in order:

1. Turn on the line switch. On some x-ray machines it is also necessary to plug the machine into a wall socket.

2.   Check the dials to verify that the current is entering the machine (some machines have both a voltmeter and milliammeter, others just one or the other).

3.   Set the milliampere regulator as required. Most techniques require the use of 10 or 15 mA.

4.   Set the kilovoltage control for the desired kilovolt peak. Most techniques require the use of between 65 and 90 kVp.

5.   Adjust the voltage regulator if the machine has one.

6.   Set the timer for the desired exposure time.

7.   Place the x-ray film packet in the patient's mouth. The film is either held in place digitally by the patient or through the use of a film holding device.

8.   Adjust the position indicating device (PID) so that the central beam of radiation is directed toward the center of the film.

9.   Pick up the timer cord and move to an area of safety (at least 6 feet away or behind the cover of structural shielding such as a lead-lined wall or partition). Press the release button and hold it down firmly until the exposure is completed.

10. Watch the needle on the milliammeter while the exposure is being made. If it fails to move or go to the proper position, it indicates a malfunction caused either by a temporarily overloaded circuit or by failure to keep a firm pressure on the timer button.

11. Remove the film from the patient's mouth after each exposure. After the final exposure, turn off the line switch and fold up the extension arm bracket as far as it will go. The tube head is finely counterbalanced in its suspension from the extension arm. This balance can be disturbed if the tube is left suspended for prolonged time periods with the extension arm stretched out.

12. As an additional precaution to prevent damage to the tube, unplug the machine at the end of each working day.

producing good radiographs

The x-rays emerging from the tube head are of many energies. The weak ones lack sufficient energy to penetrate to the film and therefore do not contribute to the film image; instead they are absorbed in the patient's skin. This is undesirable as it needlessly increases the radiation absorbed by the patient. Certain materials, especially aluminum, have the ability to absorb these "soft" undesired x-rays. This process is known as *filtration*. The beam of radiation spreads out like the spokes of a wheel as it leaves the target and emerges from the tube head. This is undesirable because it spreads the radiation to parts of the body not being x-rayed. It is important to restrict the size of the beam to the minimum size necessary to expose the film. This can be done by placing a lead diaphragm (washer) in the aperture (port) just in front of the aluminum filter disk. This process is called *collimation*. Both filtration and collimation will be discussed further in Chapter 6.

The quality of the finished radiograph, as well as the total exposure that the operator and the patient receive, is determined by several things: (1) the degree of filtration and collimation of the machine; (2) the distance of the film from the source of the radiation; (3) the speed of the film; (4) the milliamperage; (5) the kilovoltage; and (6) the exposure time. An additional influence is how the film is processed. Faulty processing diminishes the diagnostic value of the film, and often makes re-exposure necessary. This wastes time and may be dangerous to operator and patient.

There are three basic requirements for an acceptable radiograph. First, all parts of the structures radiographed must be shown on the film as close to their natural shapes and sizes as the patient's oral anatomy will permit. Distortion and superimposition of structures should be at a minimum. Second, the area examined must be shown completely, with enough surrounding tissue for the dentist to distinguish between the structures shown. Third, the film itself must be high in quality with proper density, contrast, and definition.

Density, also known as film blackening, is the amount of light transmitted through the film. The radiograph is a film negative and all photographic negatives appear darker when more light reaches the film. Thus the degree of darkening of the radiograph is increased when the amperage is increased and more x-ray photons reach the film emulsion. *Contrast*, closely related to density, refers to how sharply dark and light areas are differentiated. A film with good contrast will contain black, white, and many shades of gray. *Definition* refers to the sharpness and clarity of outline of the structures shown on the film.

variable radiation control factors

Numerous factors are involved in the exposure of radiographs. All of these factors affect the quality of the radiograph and the safety of the patient and operator. Coincidentally, the factors which improve safety also improve the quality of the radiograph. Those factors related to radiation hazards and protection are presented in the next two chapters.

Variations in the character and composition of the radiation beam have tremendous influence on the quality of the radiograph. Although the operator has little control over the variety of wavelengths in the radiation beam, there are three variables on the x-ray machine that can easily be adjusted by manipulating the controls. These variables— the milliamperage, the exposure time, and the kilovoltage—are known either as the control factors, the exposure factors, or the radiation beam factors.

The effects of all three variables are interrelated. A change in any factor involved in producing radiographs can be compensated for by adjusting one or both other factors. Distance, an additional variable factor, is not as easy to control. Whenever one of the control factors is drastically altered, one or a combination of the other factors must be proportionally altered. For example, exposure time may be decreased when milliamperage or kilovoltage is increased.

effects of variations in milliamperage

The amount of electric current used in the x-ray machine is expressed in milliamperes. The milliamperage selected by the operator determines the quantity or number of x-rays that are generated within the tube. A collateral effect is that a relation exists between milliamperage and kilovoltage. Changing the milliamperage produces slight modifications in the kilovoltage and the wavelength of the radiation beam.

The density of the radiograph is affected whenever the operator changes the milliamperage. Increasing the milliamperage increases (darkens) the density, whereas decreasing the milliamperage decreases (lightens) the density of the radiograph. To a lesser extent, slight changes in contrast occur also; usually these are not significant. Changing the milliamperage is an effective method of controlling density.

effects of variations in exposure time

Exposure time is the interval that the x-ray machine is fully activated and x-ray photons are produced. Although the principal effect of changes in exposure time is on the density of the radiograph, minor changes in contrast may also be produced. Increasing the exposure time darkens the radiograph while decreasing exposure time lightens it. Opinions differ on optimum density and contrast because visual perception varies from person to person. Some dentists may prefer lighter or darker radiographs, thus the operator must evaluate the relative effects of the various exposure factors in relation to the bone and tissue density of the patient's structures that must be penetrated

by the x-rays and make a judgment concerning which factor to increase or decrease.

Since both milliamperage and exposure time are used to regulate
the number of x-ray photons generated and have the same effect on
radiographic density, it is common practice to combine them into a
common factor *milliampere/seconds* (mAs). Both milliamperes and
exposure time are linear factors in that they are expressed in the first
power only—hence, doubling either factor also doubles the quantity
of radiation produced. Combining the milliamperage with the exposure time is the only effective way to determine the total radiation
generated. A simple formula for determining this total is mA times
exposure time equals mAs.

effects of variations in kilovoltage

The quality of the radiation (wavelength or energy of the x-ray
photons) generated by the x-ray machine is expressed in kilovoltage
or kilovoltage peak (kVp). As already stated, the more the kVp is
increased, the shorter the wavelength and the higher the energy and
penetrating power of the x-ray photons thus produced. Although the
main result of increasing the kVp is to increase the energy of the photons, a collateral effect is that the number of photons is also increased.
Thus, each exposure factor—milliamperage, exposure time, and kilovoltage—is related and each contributes to the number of x-ray photons produced. Unlike milliamperage and exposure time, kilovoltage
is an exponential factor; that is, it is expressed in powers other than
one. For practical purposes, the exposure time should be cut in half
whenever an increase of 15 kVp is made, and doubled when decreased
by 15 kVp.

Because the use of higher kVp creates high-energy photons, it is
advantageous to increase the kVp whenever the area to be examined
is thick or has great density. With experience, the radiographer can
evaluate the thickness of the patient's facial or dental structures and
determine the optimum kVp. There is no standard kVp technique
that is used in all dental offices, dental radiographs being exposed in
ranges from 45 kVp to 100 kVp.

When other exposure factors are held constant, an increase in kilovoltage peak will result in a corresponding increase in the contrast and
density of the radiograph. In order to maintain proper radiographic
contrast and density, one must reduce the mAs whenever the kVp
is increased. Since the photons generated through higher voltages
have more energy, it follows that fewer are required to expose a radiograph to desired density. However, changes in density can be more

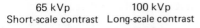

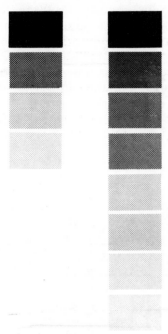

Fig. 4-1 Penetrometer tests demonstrate radiographically that a much longer contrast scale results from the use of 100-kilovolt technics. Dental radiographs at 100 kVp have longer scale contrasts. They show a marked difference compared to identical views at lower kilovoltages, having no hard "sparkle" and no chalky whites or opaque blacks. (Courtesy of General Electric, Medical Systems Division.)

effectively made by adjusting the milliampere/seconds, while changes in contrast are easiest to make by changing the kilovoltage.

Thus we see that kVp is the primary influence on image contrast (Fig. 4-1). When the differences in density between two adjacent areas of the radiograph are great, the film is said to possess *short-scale* contrast. When these differences are small, the film is said to have *long-scale* contrast. The gray tones indicate the differences in absorption of the x-ray photons by the various tissues of the oral cavity or the head. The film is *radiolucent* (dark) where the tissues are soft or thin, and *radiopaque* (white) where the tissues are thick or hard.

As a rule, the greatest degree of black-white contrast (short-scale contrast) is produced when low kilovoltage is used. The detection of caries is easier when contrast is greatest as occurs when the exposure is made in the range of 65 to 70 kVp. The higher the kVp used, the smaller is the difference between the various contrasts (long-scale contrast). With the exception of caries, the radiographic interpretation of most dental disease processes is improved with higher kVp. This brings out more shades of gray on the radiographs, thus providing more details to help the dentist in his interpretation.

Modern x-ray machines can be operated at higher kilovoltages than the older ones. There are pros and cons for employing higher kilovoltages. A distinct advantage is that the higher energy x-rays reach the film emulsion with less of them being absorbed by the intervening tissues; a disadvantage is that the exposure of tissues behind the film is increased and that more scatter radiation is produced. If the kVp used is greater than required such scatter radiation may form a fog on the film and reduce the visible contrast on the radiograph. All considered, when correctly applied, the use of higher kVp results in a slight reduction in the total amount of patient radiation dose and in a radiograph that is easier to interpret.

effects of variations in distances

The operator must take into account several distances in making x-ray exposures: the distances between the source of the x-rays on the target of the anode and the surface of the patient's skin, the distance between the x-ray source and the recording plane of the film, and the distance between the object to be x-rayed (usually the tooth) and the film. Various terms are used in dental literature to describe these distances. The terms *target-surface, anode-surface, focus-surface*, and *source-surface* are synonymous, as are *target-film, anode-film, focus-film*, and *source-film*. In this text the terms *target-surface distance* and *target-film distance* will be used.

Generally, whenever the film is positioned intraorally (within the mouth), the length of the target-surface distance depends upon the length of the position indicating device used. These PID's are classified as being short or long. All intraoral techniques require that the end of the PID should almost touch the skin—this is necessary to standardize measurements. The National Bureau of Standards Handbook 76 (1961) sets the minimum target-surface distance at 7 inches for x-ray machines operating at above 50 kVp and at 4 inches for those that operate at 50 kVp or lower. There are no maximum distances. These are governed to a certain extent by the energy of the beam. In extraoral radiography, where larger films are positioned outside the face, target-surface distances of up to 72 inches are occasionally used.

The object-film distance depends largely upon the method that is employed to hold the film in position behind the teeth. When the digital method in which the patient holds the film is used, the film is pressed against the lingual tissues as close as the oral anatomy will permit. This results in the object-film distance being shorter in the area of the crown where the tooth and film may touch than in the area opposite the root where the thickness of the bone and gingiva may cause a divergence between the long axis of the tooth and the film. The least divergence occurs in the mandibular molar areas while the greatest divergence is in the maxillary anterior areas where the palatal structures may curve sharply. With a few exceptions, most film holders are designed so that the film is held parallel to the average long axes of the teeth being x-rayed. This necessitates positioning the film sufficiently to the lingual of the teeth to avoid impinging on the supporting bone and gingival structures. This technique results in object-film distances that are often more than an inch.

The target-film distance is the sum of the target-surface and the object-film distance. In most intraoral procedures, either an 8-inch or a 16-inch distance is used. In the 8-inch technique a short PID is used and the film is positioned in direct contact with the lingual tissues, while in the 16-inch technique a longer PID is used and the film is positioned far enough from the teeth to enable it to be held parallel. These techniques will be described in detail in Chapter 11.

The length of the target-film distance is very important and has an effect on the intensity of the radiation, the amount of radiation that a patient receives, and the dimensional accuracy of the image produced on the radiograph (the latter is also affected by the object-film distance).

The intensity of the radiation beam varies inversely to the square of the target-film distance (Fig. 4-2). This is based on the inverse

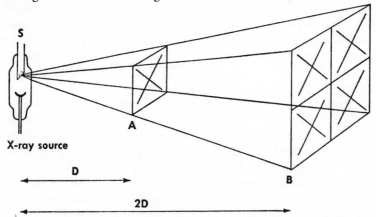

Fig. 4-2 Relationship of distance to the area covered by x-rays emanating from an x-ray tube. Photons emerging from the tube travel in straight lines and diverge from each other. The areas covered by the photons at any two points are proportional to each other as the square of the distances measured from the points to the source of radiation. (From Wuehrmann, Arthur H., and Manson-Hing, Lincoln R. *Dental Radiography*, 2d ed. St. Louis: The C. V. Mosby Co., 1969.)

square law, which states that the intensity of light varies inversely as the square of the distance from its source. Since the x-ray photons emerging from the tube travel in straight lines and diverge from each other, it follows that the intensity of the beam is reduced unless a corresponding increase is made in one or a combination of the exposure factors. Such changes in exposure factors are essential to maintaining optimum film density. Because milliamperage and time are the main factors influencing film density the following formula can be used to determine the mAs-distance relationship:

$$\frac{\text{Original mAs}}{\text{New mAs}} = \frac{\text{Original distance}^2}{\text{New distance}^2}$$

For example, if a film of the same speed were used in two exposures and the mA and the kVp were left unchanged it would only be necessary to increase the exposure time when the target-film distance is doubled. In that event, by applying the formula given, the exposure time must be increased fourfold. Tripling the distance would require a ninefold increase. This and all further increases in mAs are based on this formula in which the distances are squared.

The exposure dose that the patient receives decreases proportionally as the target-film distance increases. When distance is doubled, the exposure dose is reduced to one-fourth. In actuality, this would not happen because it is necessary to change the other exposure factors to maintain adequate film density. However, skin exposure is slightly reduced at greater target-film distance because less tissue falls within the diverging beam of radiation. The x-ray photons diverge to form this beam of radiation; the closer the tube is brought to the face, the more the beam diverges behind the skin area and the greater is the area of irradiated tissue (Fig. 4-3).

Of greater significance than the slight decrease in exposure dose is that the quality of the radiographic image improves whenever the target-film distance is increased. Dimensional distortion and magnification are less and sharpness of detail (definition) is greater. The decrease in dimensional distortion is largely attributable to the use of film holders that keep the film parallel with the teeth. Film holders form an integral part of the 16-inch target-film technique. When the 8-inch target-film distance is used, the outer, more divergent rays tend to magnify the image. The closer the target is to the teeth, the greater the magnification. As the distance from the target is lengthened, the image is produced by the more central rays of the beam which are more parallel to each other and consequently decrease the magnification. Although image sharpness is also affected by movement of the

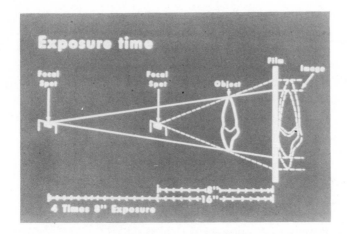

Fig. 4-3 Comparison of 8 in. and 16 in. target-film (T/F) distance. The image is enlarged when the T/F distance is shortened and the object (tooth) to film distance is held constant. Ideally, the distance from the target to the object should be as long as practical and the distance from the object to the film should be as short as possible. When using the 16 in. T/F distance, the exposure time must be lengthened approximately four times that required at 8 in. (From Updegrave, William J. *New Horizons in Periapical and Interproximal Radiographs.* Elgin, Illinois: The Rinn Corporation, 1971.)

patient, the size of the grains in the film emulsion, the size of the focal spot, and the object-film distance, increasing the target-film distance reduces the fuzzy outline (called a penumbra) which is around all radiographic images.

More dentists are using the longer target-film distances than ever before. The acceptance of the 16-inch target-film distance was delayed until film manufacturers started to produce films so sensitive that they could be exposed in a mere fraction of the time required by the older films. At greater target-film distances the patient receives less radiation, but so does the film. The quadrupled exposure time required when the distance was doubled resulted in such long exposures that patient movement or film slippage was likely to occur. Another factor which made longer target-film distances practical was the development of more powerful x-ray machines with electronic timers.

Most operators readily memorize the exposure factors they need to know for the particular technique they are using. Several excellent charts or conversion tables are available through the manufacturers of the films or the x-ray equipment. These show at a glance how much exposure time is required for a film of any given film speed when used with all possible combinations of exposure time, milliamperage, and peak kilovoltage. Many operators fasten these charts beside the control panel. Some recent x-ray machine models incorporate the most commonly used film speeds and other exposure factors into the dial of the control panel. In that case the operator only has to set the pointer to the desired combination for a film of a given speed; all the rest is done automatically when the timer release button is depressed.

bibliography

Ennis, Leroy M., Berry, Harrison M., and Phillips, James E. *Dental Roentgenology*, 6th ed. Philadelphia: Lea & Febiger, 1967.

Kinsman, Simon, and Alcox, Ray W. *Radiation Hygiene in Dental Radiography*, Sacramento: State of California, Department of Public Health, Bureau of Radiological Health, 1970.

Peterson, Shailer. *Clinical Dental Hygiene*, 3d ed. St. Louis: The C. V. Mosby Co., 1968.

Updegrave, William J. *New Horizons in Periapical and Interproximal Radiography*, Elgin, Ill.: Rinn Corporation, 1971.

Wainwright, William Ward. *Dental Radiography*, New York: McGraw-Hill Book Co., 1965.

Wilkins, Esther M. *Clinical Practice of the Dental Hygienist*, 3d ed. Philadelphia: Lea & Febiger, 1971.

Wuehrmann, Arthur H., and Manson-Hing, Lincoln R. *Dental Radiology*, 2d ed. St. Louis: The C. V. Mosby Co., 1969.

X-Ray Generation and Radiographic Principles in Dentistry, Milwaukee: General Electric Company, Technical Services, X-Ray Department.

X-Rays in Dentistry, Rochester, N.Y.: Eastman Kodak Co., 1972.

5
effects
of radiation exposure

general effects of radiation

As we have said, radiation may occur naturally or be man-made.
Cosmic rays are present in the universe, and radiation is also emitted
continuously by radioactive elements in the earth. These forms,
called background radiations, account for about a third of the total
radiation received by persons living in our advanced technological
society. Aside from the occasional hazard of overexposure to the
sun or of unknowingly being near a deposit of radioactive minerals,
background radiations are of small concern to us.

What concerns us more are the man-made radiations—emissions
from industrial atomic waste, from military testing of atomic weap-
ons, and from certain commercial products. Of special concern are
radiations used in industry, medicine, and dentistry. These account
for some 90 percent of the man-made radiations to which the general
public is exposed.

Any exposure to radiation has at least a little biological effect on
the exposed person. Unfortunately, we do not yet fully understand
all these effects or their future consequences. Scientists believe that
some of these effects are cumulative, especially if exposure is too
great and the intervals between exposures too frequent for the body
cells to repair themselves. Unless the damage is too severe or the
subject is in extremely poor health, most body cell (somatic cells)
recovery rate is almost 75 percent during the first twenty-four hours;
after that repair continues at the same rate. Thus it is good practice,
before using x-rays, to ask whether the patient works around radiation or has had other recent x-rays. In some cases a delay may be
advisable.

In determining whether or not an exposure is potentially harmful, the radiographer should consider especially the quantity and the duration of the exposure and which body area is to be irradiated. Continued exposure over prolonged periods alters the ability of the genetic cells (eggs and sperm) to reproduce normally. Although present evidence indicates that chromosome damage is cumulative and genetic cells cannot repair themselves, thus resulting in possible sterilization of the radiated person or in the altering of the genetic material in the reproductive cells so that mutations (abnormalities) may be produced in future generations, using lead aprons and proper safety techniques will protect the patient from any conceivable damage. The benefits of dental radiographs far outweigh the minor risks to patient and radiographer.

cell sensitivity to radiation exposure

The sensitivity of both somatic and genetic cells to radiation exposure differs enormously from person to person. Just as some persons are almost immune to certain diseases or can stay in the sun without becoming ill or burning, so people vary in their reactions to radiation exposure. Age, general health, and the type of cell exposed— its location, chemical composition, blood supply, rate of metabolism or reproductive activity—also play a major role in cell sensitivity.

The terms *radiosensitive* and *radioresistant* are used to describe the degree of susceptibility of various body tissues to radiation. All cells contain a nucleus and cytoplasm that control cellular activity. This activity can under certain circumstances be impaired by exposure to radiation. Generally, cells with high metabolic activity or those with a short lifespan that are involved in continuous cell division are extremely radiosensitive. Highly specialized or mature cells are relatively radioresistant. Thus the genetic (reproductive) cells and the somatic cells in the blood-forming tissues are most radiosensitive. In descending order of radiosensitivity are the rest of the somatic cells—young bone cells, lymphatic cells, glandular epithelial cells, epithelial cells lining the alimentary tract and the body cavities, the epithelial cells of the skin, and muscle cells. Nerve cells and mature bone cells are among the most radioresistant.

Oral structures, with their high proportion of bone, are quite radioresistant. Moreover, in dental radiation, exposure is limited to this very small area, and the amount of radiation is small. Therefore dental radiation may be considered quite safe. Specific measures for making radiation safe for both patient and operator are described in the next chapter.

the mechanics of biological damage

As we have seen in Chapter 2, high-energy radiations have the ability to detach and remove certain subatomic electric charges from the complex atoms that make up the molecules of body tissues. This process, known as ionizing radiation, creates an electrical imbalance within the normally stable cells. Because disturbed cellular atoms or molecules generally attempt to regain electrical stability, they often accept the first available opposite electrical charge. In such cases the cells that contain these now altered atoms or molecules may undergo undesirable chemical or physical changes, becoming incompatible with the surrounding body tissues. During ionization the delicate cell balance of the cell structure is altered and changes may take place that may damage or destroy the cell. Obviously, we have no way of knowing how such mutations will progress, but we can assume that such altered cell structures are undesirable. For this reason the radiographer must always be alert to use all possible skill to avoid exposing the body to unnecessary ionizing radiation.

Numerous theories on how ionizing radiation produces intercellular damage have been advanced. The two most accepted are: (1) the direct hit or target theory, and (2) the indirect action or poison water theory.

According to the direct hit theory, x-ray photons collide with cell walls and break them apart, causing physical damage to the large molecules of body tissue (Fig. 5–1). But, in fact, most x-ray photons probably pass through the cell with little or no damage. A healthy cell can easily repair any minor damage. Besides, the body contains so many cells that the destruction of a single cell or small group of cells has no observable effect.

The indirect action theory is based on the assumption that radiation can cause chemical damage to the cell by ionizing the water within it. Since about 80 percent of body weight is water, and ionization can dissociate water into hydrogen and hydroxyl radical, the

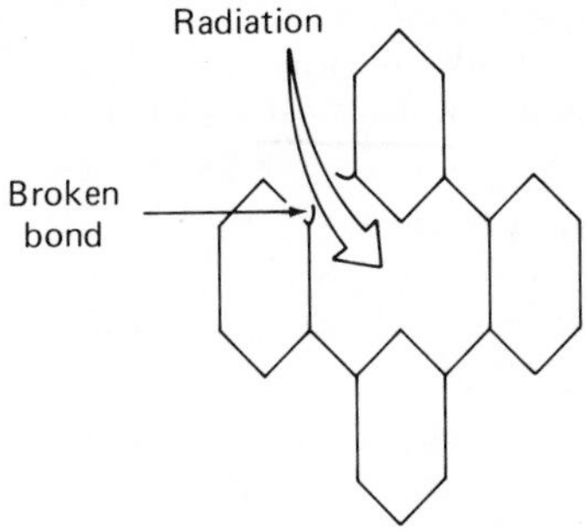

Radiation

Broken
bond

Fig. 5–1 Radiation breaks the bonds connecting atoms in molecules, thus producing harmful effects. A living cell consists mostly of water. Breakdown products of water can form hydrogen peroxide (H_2O_2), which can break down protein. (From Stickland, William D., and Baker, Benjamin R. *Dental Assisting*, V, Clinical Sciences, 2d ed. Chapel Hill, University of North Carolina Press, 1971.)

theory proposes that a new chemical called hydrogen peroxide could be formed under certain conditions. This strong chemical acts as a poison to the body, causing cellular dysfunction. Fortunately, when the water is broken down during ionizing radiation, the ions have a strong tendency to recombine immediately to form water again instead of seeking out new combinations. This tendency holds cellular damage to a minimum. Under ordinary circumstances, even when a new chemical is formed, other cells that are not affected can take over the functions of the damaged cells until recovery takes place. Only in extreme instances, where massive irradiation has taken place, will entire body areas be destroyed or death result.

Much about radiation effects remains to be discovered. Moreover, much of our radiation research is conducted with experimental animals much smaller than we are. Not all species have the same radiosensitivity. Conceivably, future research may demonstrate that man is not nearly as susceptible to radiation damage as we now believe. But until we have evidence, it is only common sense to improve radiographic safety techniques in every possible way.

studies on radiation exposure protection

As early as 1902 some studies were undertaken to determine the effect of radiation exposure on the body and to consider setting limits on radiation exposure. The International Commission on Radiation Protection was formed in 1928, and in 1929 the National Council on Radiation Protection and Measurements (NCRP) was created in the United States. The American Dental Association (ADA), through its various committees and affiliated organizations, works closely with all organizations interested in radiation safety. It will send its publications to those who write for them.

Research on the effects of radiation and on radiation hygiene procedures sped forward when scientists and the public became alarmed in the early 1950's over possible radiation effects produced by atomic testing. The U. S. Atomic Energy Commission promptly adopted the strict NCRP recommendations and incorporated them into rules and regulations published in the Federal Register. Many organizations studied the various aspects of radiation safety and production simultaneously, but not necessarily from the same viewpoint. All known forms of radiation were studied, but the major effort was directed toward finding out what levels of radiation could safely be tolerated and accumulated.

As a result of all these studies the NCRP proposed two sets of limits, one for dentists and dental personnel and the other for patients. It suggested that patient exposures be kept at a minimum consistent with clinical requirements, but left the limits to the professional judgment of the dentist. The maximum limits were set higher for workers than for the public, but the suggested limits of maximum permissible accumulated exposure for both groups were purposely set lower than it was believed the body could safely accept.

Over the years there has been a constant downward revision of the acceptable limits which are now about seven hundred times smaller than those originally proposed in 1902. Many aspects of tissue damage from radiation, especially the duration of the latent period (see definition in next section) are still not clearly understood. It is interesting to note that the statute of limitations does not apply to radiation injuries for this reason; that is, a patient may sue the dentist at any time for radiation damage he believes he received as a result of dental x-rays, even years after the radiation was given.

Although the NCRP and similar organizations have no legal status, their suggestions and recommendations are highly regarded. Many regulatory bodies have used them to formulate legislation controlling the use of radiation in the dental office. Two publications are recommended for obtaining additional information concerning radiation protection: (1) NCRP Report No. 35, *Dental X-Ray Protection*, Washington, D.C.: 1970 ($1.50), and (2) NCRP Report No. 39, *Basic Radiation Protection Criteria*, Washington, D.C.: 1971 ($2.00).

radiation measurement terminology

It will be useful to define a few terms used in this and subsequent chapters. These and other terms also appear in the glossary.

Roentgen (R): The unit of exposure to radiation. This is the exposure required to produce in air 2.58 times 10^4 coulomb of ions of either sign per kilogram of air (Fig. 5-2). A simpler definition of the roentgen is that it is the amount of x or gamma radiation required to ionize one cc. of air at standard conditions of pressure and temperature.

Rad: A special unit of absorbed dose equal to 100 ergs per gram of tissue. For x-rays, the rad is numerically the same as the roentgen.

Rem: The unit of dose equivalent. For radiation protection purposed, the number of rems of x-rays may be considered equal to the number of rads or the number of roentgen.

Absorbed Dose: The energy imparted to matter by ionizing particles per unit of mass of irradiated material at the place of interest. The special unit of absorbed dose is the *rad.*

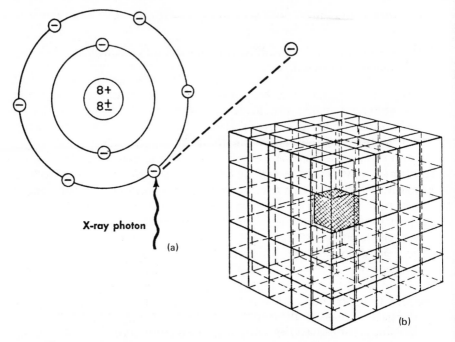

Fig. 5–2 Schematic representation. (a) Ionization of an oxygen atom; (b) 1 cm cube of air surrounded by an infinite amount of air. (From Wuehrmann, Arthur H., and Manson-Hing, Lincoln R. *Dental Radiography*, 2d ed. St. Louis: The C. V. Mosby Co., 1969.)

Dose Equivalent: A quantity used for radiation protection purposes that expresses on a common scale for all radiations the irradiation incurred by exposed persons. It is defined as the product of absorbed dose in rads and certain modifying factors. The unit of dose equivalent is the *rem*.

Maximum Permissible Dose Equivalent: For radiation protection purposes, the maximum dose equivalent that a person or body part is allowed to receive in a stated period of time. For whole-body radiation this is currently set at 5 rems per year for radiation workers.

Exposure: A measure of ionization produced in air by x or gamma radiation. The special unit of exposure is the *roentgen*.

Exposure Rate: The exposure per unit of time.

Radiation (ionizing): Radiation capable of producing ions directly or indirectly by interaction with matter.

Threshold Exposure: The minimum exposure that will produce a detectable degree of any given effect.

Erythema Exposure: The amount of radiation required to produce temporary redness of the skin.

Latent Period: The period of time between exposure to radiation and clinically observable symptoms.

radiation measurement and measuring devices

The problem of radiation measurement is complicated because radiation measuring instruments can measure only radiation received at skin surface but not that within the body. One may attach a measuring device to the skin surface at one side of the face to determine the entrance dose (also called skin or exposure dose) and attach another meter to the other side of the face to determine the exit dose. However, one may only estimate the depth dose, or amount of exposure between entrance and exit, by considering such factors as the distance from the point of entrance or exit, the quality of the radiation, and the types of intervening tissues. The same holds true when attempting to estimate radiation to genetic tissues. The size and sex of the patient make a difference, the gonads of a child being closer to the source of radiation than those of an adult, and the female organs being better protected by the abdominal structures than those of the male. Some reports state that only 0.0005 R are received by the patient's genetic tissues during a routine full-mouth radiographic examination made under optimal conditions, or that an operator can expose 300 high-speed films per week at little risk to himself. But such figures are educated calculations, because radiation itself cannot be measured in all body areas.

Although effects of radiation on patients are difficult to determine and depth doses difficult to measure, it is possible to measure accurately the amount of radiation on a film badge or similar device. These will be described in the next chapter.

specific effects of radiation

Observable radiation effects are classified as short- or long-term effects. Short-term effects are generally caused by acute doses in which the radiation is delivered either to a specific area or to a large body area in a very short period of time. An acute overexposure may be accidental, as in the case of the failure of an atomic experiment, or it may be deliberately and meticulously induced as a treatment for a malignancy. The latent period is generally fairly short in acute exposures and grows progressively shorter as the dose level is raised.

Erythema, a rash-like reddening of the skin is the earliest and most commonly observable effect. It may appear in only hours or after several weeks. Aside from erythema, brief whole body doses in the range of 50 to 100 R may produce vomiting, diarrhea, and general malaise. No recent records exist of such occurrence in dental practice. Massive acute exposures in the range of 400 to 500 R can result in death.

Long-term effects of radiation may manifest themselves years after the original exposure. Such delayed effects may be the result of previous acute massive exposures or from chronic often repeated smaller exposures over a period of time. The latent period in such chronic exposures is totally unpredictable. Observable effects of long-term exposure include loss of hair, splitting of nails, cataract formation, and certain neoplasms. Other effects like lifespan shortening, embryological effects, genetic effects, internal carcinogenic effects, and blood changes are more difficult to detect. Symptoms of leukemia and cancer often remain undetected for prolonged periods.

No one has ever demonstrated that cancer in a patient has ever been caused by dental radiography but many dentists have suffered from cancer of the hand caused by holding x-ray films in the mouths of patients. The lens of the eye is also a tissue that is sensitive to radiation. Unfortunately, most dental x-rays are directed toward the vicinity of the eyes. Although dental radiations are not known to have caused cataracts in patients, we should minimize x-ray exposure to the eye as much as possible. The new lead-lined PID's that limit the size of the beam accomplish this.

Special consideration should be given to protect young women in the reproductive ages from embryological effects during radiographic procedures. The fetus, particularly in the first trimester of human pregnancy, is composed of rapidly growing unspecialized tissues. For this reason, exposures should be kept to an absolute minimum during this time and protective lead aprons should always be draped over the patient.

guides for maintaining safe radiation levels

The NCRP developed radiation protection guidelines (also referred to as Maximum Permissible Doses) for the protection of radiation workers and the general public. The guides represent doses far below those at which any effects have ever been observed. The general public is permitted 1/10 the exposure permitted radiation workers. This was done because workers represent only a small fraction of the total population, and it was believed that if they suffer greater genetic

damage than the general population, the damaged hereditary material
will be so diluted in the general population that it will not cause a
disastrous mutation level. Radiation necessary for medical or dental
diagnostic purposes is not counted in the permissible amounts of
radiation.

Permissible exposure limits for dentists and dental personnel are
the same as for other radiation workers. According to these guidelines the accumulated dosage may not exceed 3 rems for a 13-week
period or 5 rems for a calendar year. There is no established weekly
limit but the average exposure should be limited to 0.1 rem. There
are some exceptions to these guidelines; the skin of the whole body,
the hands and forearms, and the feet and ankles may receive larger
exposure doses. Another exception is for persons under 18 years of
age; a federal law prohibits employment of such persons for work
that involves radiation.

The formula 5 times age of the radiographer minus 18 [expressed
5(N–18) equals the maximum permissible accumulated exposure in
rems] is used to determine the previous accumulated occupational
exposure of an individual if not known. It shall be assumed that he
has already received the full dose permitted each previous year. The
N in the formula equals the age in years and is greater than 18. The
reports from any film badge service are the most reliable permanent
records of accumulated exposure. If a worker's film badge indicates
that the average weekly levels are frequently exceeded, there is jus-
tifiable cause for concern. All techniques should be reviewed for
errors and the x-ray machine should be tested for leakage.

Guides are also established for students. In learning to expose
radiographs, students should not expose more than one full-mouth
series on each other. These radiographs must serve a diagnostic purpose and be interpreted by a dentist. Additional practice on patients
(if permissible by state law) can be accomplished by the use of referred patients, provided the radiographs are given to their dentist
for diagnostic interpretation.

Presently there are no legal limits to the radiation to which the
public may be exposed. The limitation to 1/10 the exposure permitted radiation workers is a guide and very few persons are likely to
receive even half this amount. Studies indicate that the average person
in an advanced technological society receives approximately equal
parts of natural background and man-made radiations. The NCRP
has recommended that the total genetic dose of radiation received
by the general population during the first 30 years of life should not
exceed 10 rems of man-made radiation. Each individual may accumu-
late another 10 rems in each succeeding decade. The radiation bank

Radiation bank
deposits

Radiation exposure of genetic tissue

		and
	$3.33	$3.33
$10.00	more	every 10
at birth	at 30	years, i.e.,
	years	at 40 years,

10 roentgens from birth to 30 years
to the general population from
man-made radiations

50 years,
60 years,
70 years,
etc.

Maximum permissible dose

Withdrawals

Chest film — 0.001 roentgens (or 1 milliroentgen) — $0.001

GI Series — 1 roentgen (1,000 milliroentgens) — $1.00

Barium enema — 1 roentgen (2 roentgens in the female) — $1.00

Set of dental radiographs (adult male-20 films)

old-time machine and slow film
0.3 roentgens (or 300 milliroentgens) — $0.30

modern machine and ultrafast film
0.001 roentgens (or 1 milliroentgen) — $0.001

Panoramic dental radiograph — 0.001 roentgens — $0.001

Natural radiation — 4 roentgens per 30 years — add 0.5 roentgens at 5,000 feet elevation

Radium dial wrist watch — 0.5 roentgens per 15 years — $0.50

Fall-Out — 0.1 roentgens per 30 years at the 1960 rate — $0.10

8 Sets of dental radiographs — modern machine and ultrafast film
0.02 roentgens (8 sets are ample to carry a patient from birth to 30 years) — $0.02

(Fig. 5–3) in which dollars are used to represent roentgens gives a realistic portrayal of the sources of radiation to which a person may be exposed during such periods. To translate these statistics into more meaningful terms, a patient in a medical office may receive up to 1 rem of whole-body exposure from a gastrointestinal series of radiographs, but a dental patient receives only 0.001 rem of whole-body radiation from a complete 20-film set of radiographs if modern techniques and high-speed films are used. Such procedures fall well within the guidelines for radiation safety.

All those using dental x-ray equipment must be aware of the rigid standards and regulations established by city, county, state, and federal agencies and must be prepared to observe them. The California legislature requires that dental workers must pass a radiation safety examination before they can expose radiographs; similar legislation is considered in other states. In some instances, city and county regulations are stricter than those imposed by the states.

Some patients have heard highly exaggerated stories concerning radiation—a few based on facts now outdated and many on misinformation and rumor. Occasionally, a patient is reluctant to submit to any form of x-radiation. His objections can generally be overcome if the dentist, dental hygienist, or dental assistant takes the time to educate him. Thus it is doubly important that anyone who practices radiography be thoroughly informed.

bibliography

Baker, Benjamin R., and Strickland, William D. *Dental Assisting,* Course V, Clinical Sciences, 2d ed. Chapel Hill: University of North Carolina Press, 1971.

Kinsman, Simon, and Alcox, Ray W. *Radiation Hygiene in Dental Radiography,* Sacramento: State of California, Department of Public Health, Bureau of Radiological Health, 1970.

National Council on Radiation Protection and Measurements, NCRP Report No. 35, *Dental X-Ray Protection,* Washington, D.C.: NCRP, 1970.

National Council on Radiation Protection and Measurements, NCRP Report No. 39, *Basic Radiation Protection Criteria,* Washington, D.C.: NCRP, 1971.

Fig. 5–3 The radiation bank. (From Wainwright, William Ward. *Dental Radiography.* New York: McGraw-Hill Book Company, 1965. Copyright © 1965 by McGraw-Hill Inc. Used with permission of McGraw-Hill Book Company.)

O'Brien, Richard C. *Dental Radiography*, 2d ed. Philadelphia: W. B. Saunders Co., 1972.

Peterson, Shailer. *Clinical Dental Hygiene*, 3d ed. St. Louis: The C. V. Mosby Co., 1968.

Richardson, Richard E., and Barton, Roger E. *The Dental Assistant,* 4th ed. New York: McGraw-Hill Book Co., 1970.

Wainwright, William Ward. *Dental Radiology*, New York: McGraw-Hill Book Co., 1965.

Wuehrmann, Arthur H., and Manson-Hing, Lincoln R. *Dental Radiology,* 2d ed. St. Louis: The C. V. Mosby Co., 1969.

6

radiation protection
and monitoring

professional concern and responsibility

Any radiation exposure carries a potential for biological damage to the patient and operator, however slight. The dentist shares the public's concern over the effects of needless or excessive exposure to radiation. Since the hazard increases with the amount of radiation, everything must be done to keep radiation doses as low as possible.

The use of outdated and malfunctioning equipment, the absence of protective shielding, and carelessness or ignorance on the part of the operator all contribute to too-high dosages. The dentist has the obligation to safeguard everyone in his practice by eliminating these sources of trouble. If necessary, he must make structural changes in the walls of the operatories and replace or modify his equipment. He must also instruct or supervise all who have access to the x-ray units. In fact, the dentist is *legally* responsible for all acts or services performed in his office. For this reason and to avoid injury to the patient or operator, x-ray films should be exposed only under the direct supervision of the dentist or a qualified instructor.

radiation safety legislation

The Tenth Amendment gives the states the constitutional authority to regulate health. Because many federal agencies are involved in the development and use of atomic energy, the Federal Government has preempted the control of radiation. Certain provisions of the Constitution and Public Law 86–373 have enabled the states to assume this preempted power and pass laws that spell out radiation safety measures to protect the patient, the operator, or anyone (the general

public) near the source of radiation from indiscriminate use of ionizing radiation. In fact, even counties and cities have passed ordinances
to protect their citizens from radiation hazards. Several states and a
few localities require periodic inspection or monitoring of the equipment and its surroundings. Many are considering further laws to
provide for monitoring and to set minimum standards for x-ray operators.

Since the laws concerning radiation control vary greatly, each
person working with x-rays is urged to become familiar with the
major provisions of his own state or local radiation code and observe
its requirements. Regardless of laws, failure to observe safety procedures cannot be justified morally. Many excellent booklets and articles
on radiation safety and radiation hygiene methods are available.
Especially recommended are NCRP Reports No. 35 and 39 that are
available at nominal cost. These were mentioned in the previous
chapter and listed in the bibliography. Another excellent booklet,
Radiation Protection in Dental Practice, is published by the Department of Public Health of the State of California. This booklet is free
and is a valuable guide for establishing radiation safety programs in
dental practices.

radiation safety terminology

The following terms are important in radiation control:

Primary Beam (Primary Radiation): The original radiation that
emanates from the focal spot on the tube of the x-ray unit. It leaves
the tube head through an aperture behind the PID (cone) and travels
in a cone-shaped path, becoming constantly larger as the distance from
the focal spot (on the target) increases. Although this beam is composed of x-ray photons of various wavelengths, only the shorter waves
are needed to produce radiographs. This beam is most dangerous to
the patient in often repeated exposures.

Useful Beam (Useful Radiation): That part of the primary beam
that is permitted to emerge from the housing of the tube and is limited
by the aperture, filters, lead diaphragm (collimeter), or other collimating device such as a lead-lined PID or a scatter guard (a circular
lead device) inside an open-ended cone. The size of the useful beam
of x-radiation can be determined by the size of the aperture in the
tube housing or by the shape of the opening in the collimeter. This
opening should not be any larger than necessary to produce a beam

big enough to expose all parts of the film. According to the recommendations of the American Academy of Dental Radiology, the diameter of the useful beam should not exceed 2-3/4 inches at the tip of the PID.

Secondary Radiation: The radiation given off by any matter being irradiated with x-rays. This new form of radiation is created the moment the primary beam comes into contact with matter. During dental x-ray procedures it originates mainly in the soft tissues of the face, the soft and hard tissues of the patient's head, the plastic materials of the cone (PID), and the filters. During this reaction, the energy of the primary radiation is diminished and transformed into energy of lower wavelength.

Scatter Radiation: The radiation that has been deflected from its path by impact during its passage through matter. This form of secondary radiation (the terms secondary and scatter radiation are often used interchangeably) is emitted or deflected in all directions by the tissues of the patient's head during radiation. It then travels to all parts of the body and to adjacent areas of the room. That is why protective shielding is desirable for the operator and why the patient should be draped with a lead apron. The possibility of biological damage from secondary or scatter radiation must not be taken lightly. Though seldom in the path of the primary beam, the operator can be injured by exposure to deflected rays unless protected by adequate structural shielding, or movable lead-lined screens. Scatter radiation presents the most serious danger to the operator.

Leakage Radiation: A form of radiation that bounces off the target inside the tube and escapes in all directions through the protective shielding of the tube and tube head. Most modern x-rays have well protected tubes and tube heads, but occasionally leakage occurs, especially at the points where the electrical connections enter. The two areas where the tube head is attached to the yoke are particularly susceptible to leakage. Such leakage may be in any or all directions. Because it is usually unsuspected and can only be detected by using a special film pack or by a radiation survey, it can be very dangerous.

Filter: Absorbing material (usually aluminum) placed in the path of the beam of radiation in order to remove the more absorbable components (the longer wavelengths).

Filtration: The preferential absorption of the less penetrating components of the polychromatic x-ray beam by passage of the beam

through a sheet of material called a filter. In the dental x-ray machine, these filters are disks of pure aluminum that vary in thickness.
These filters may be sealed into the tube head or inserted into the
port where the PID attaches. Pure aluminum or its equivalent will
not hinder the passage of high-energy photons but will absorb the
low-energy photons. The latter do not contribute to the radiographic
image; in fact, they decrease its density. However, they are harmful
to the patient because they are absorbed by his skin and increase his
exposure (Fig. 6–1).

   Inherent Filtration: Filtration produced by the internal barriers
to the passage of the x-rays from the focal spot to the external surface
of the tube housing. These barriers include the tube wall, the insulating oil, and the air surrounding the tube. All x-ray units have some
built-in filtration. Most contain the equivalent of 0.5 to 3.0 mm. of
pure aluminum—the newer x-ray machines have the most inherent
filtration.

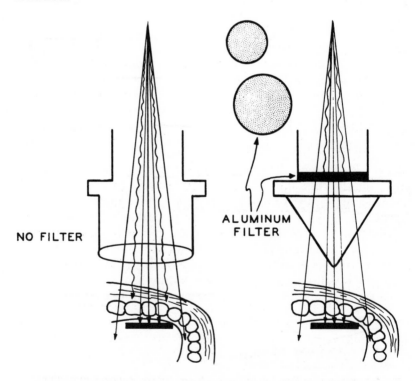

Fig. 6–1 Effect of filtration on skin exposure. (From *Radiation Protection in
Dental Practice*. Sacramento: State of California, Department of Public Health,
Bureau of Radiological Health, 1968.)

Added Filtration: Filtration placed outside the tube head. When the inherent filtration is not sufficient to meet present safety standards, a disk of aluminum of the appropriate thickness can be inserted between the port of the tube head and the PID.

Total Filtration: The sum of the inherent and added filtration expressed in mm. of aluminum equivalent. Present safety standards require an equivalent of 1.5 mm. aluminum for x-ray machines operating in ranges below 70 kVp and a minimum of 2.5 mm. aluminum for machines operating at or above 70 kVp.

Collimator: A diaphragm or tubular device made of radioresistant material (usually lead) designed to define the dimensions of the useful beam.

Collimation: The control of the size and shape of the useful beam. The most common form of collimation in dental radiography is to insert a lead diaphragm or washer at the base of the PID (Fig. 6-2).

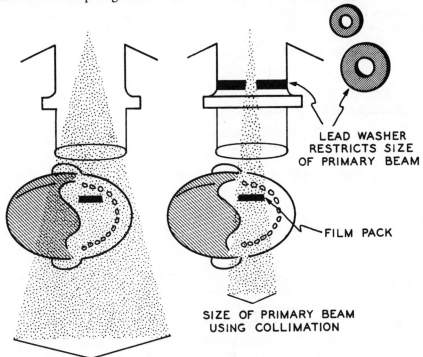

LEAD WASHER
RESTRICTS SIZE
OF PRIMARY BEAM

FILM PACK

SIZE OF PRIMARY BEAM
USING COLLIMATION

SIZE OF PRIMARY BEAM
WITHOUT COLLIMATION

Fig. 6-2 Effect of collimation on primary beam. (From *Radiation Protection in Dental Practices*. Sacramento: State of California, Department of Public Health, Bureau of Radiological Health, 1968.)

Other forms of collimation include the cylindrical scatter guards in open-ended plastic PID's and the lead-lined PID's. Although collimators can be placed in the old type pointed plastic cones, they are not as safe as the newer open-ended PID's. Not only is it impossible to attach scatter guards or line the pointed cones, but the x-rays collide with the plastic material of the cone and harmful secondary radiation is produced.

Controlled Area: A defined area in which the occupational exposure of personnel to radiation is under the supervision of the radiation protection supervisor. The dental office is designated as a controlled area; a public hallway or traffic corridor through a dental office is not so considered if used by the public.

Radiation Protection Supervisor: The person directly responsible for radiation protection. In the dental office it is usually the dentist.

Half-Value Layer: The thickness of a specified substance that, when introduced into the path of a given beam of radiation, reduces the exposure rate by one-half (Fig. 6–3).

Protective Barrier: A barrier of radiation absorbing materials, used to reduce radiation exposure.

Primary Protective Barrier: A barrier sufficient to attenuate the useful beam to the required degree.

Secondary Protective Barrier: Barrier sufficient to attenuate stray radiation to the required degree.

Structural Shielding: The protection afforded by structural materials.

radiation protection measures for operator
and patient

Since the dangers of overexposure to radiation were first recognized, many safeguards have been devised. Some of these safeguards, such as filtration, collimation, and protective shielding, are mechanical; others are technical. Some of these radiation safety techniques protect primarily the patient; others protect primarily the operator. Generally, both patient and operator benefit by them.

One of the cardinal principles in radiography is to use the least radiation needed to perform the task. Another important rule is never to hold the film for the patient or stabilize the tube head or the PID. Holding the tube head subjects the operator to possible exposure from

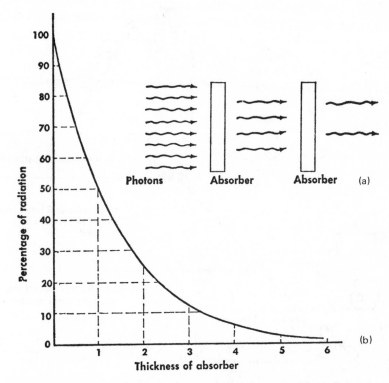

Fig. 6–3 (a) Diagram showing the effect of two half-value layers of absorbing material on a monochromatic beam of x-ray photons. (b) Graph showing the exponential curve of x-ray absorption. (From Wuehrmann, Arthur H., and Manson-Hing, Lincoln R. *Dental Radiology*, 2d ed. St. Louis: The C. V. Mosby Co., 1969.)

leakage radiation, and holding the PID places the hand right in the path of the primary beam. At this spot the radiation is 4,000 times greater than at a distance of six feet.

The operator should always stand as far as possible—at least six feet—from the source of the radiation unless he is protected by shielding. The potency of the x-radiation diminishes the further the x-rays travel (Fig. 6–4). A careless operator who stands close to the patient while making an exposure can receive a large amount of secondary or scatter radiation.

Lead-lined walls, thick or specially constructed partitions between the rooms, or specially constructed lead screens or shields afford excellent protection for the operator. The lead screens or shields contain a radiation resistant glass through which the operator looks at the patient and the dials on the control panel during exposure. When

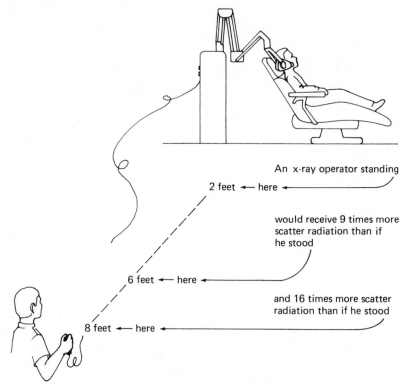

2 feet ← here ←

An x-ray operator standing

would receive 9 times more scatter radiation than if he stood

6 feet ← here ←

and 16 times more scatter radiation than if he stood

8 feet ← here ←

Fig. 6–4 Distance is an effective means of reducing exposure from scatter radiation. (From *Radiation Protection in Dental Practices.* Sacramento: State of California, Department of Public Health, Bureau of Radiological Health, 1968.)

the dental office is not equipped with such shielding, an extra-long timer cord can be used to enable the operator to step outside the operatory while making the exposure. In the absence of shielding, the safest place for the operator to stand is from 45 to 90 degrees out of the primary beam, behind the bulkiest part of the patient's head. The head thus absorbs most of the primary beam and much of the scatter radiation. All persons not directly concerned with the x-ray exposure should leave the room, and care must be taken not to accidentally expose persons who are passing by. Some states require the use of a lead apron over the abdominal area. Even if not legally required, this is important, especially for women in the first trimester of pregnancy and in young adults.

Another radiation safeguard is the use of the largest film that can be placed comfortably in the patient's mouth, so that fewer films and exposures are needed. However, this is not always practical.

Sometimes smaller films are needed to prevent bending which distorts the image. Use of film with an ASA speed of D or better (extra-fast) means shorter exposure times, too. Usually, following the processing technique recommended by the film manufacturer will reduce unnecessary exposures due to retakes of radiographs that were spoiled by under- or over-development.

equipment modifications for safety

Some older x-ray machines lack adequate filtration and collimation. Their mechanical timers are not accurate enough to measure the short exposure times used with high-speed films. Thus they often fail to meet safety standards. Even though some states are not as radiation safety conscious as others, some of these machines should be replaced. Others can be modified to make them safer and easier to control.

The addition of aluminum disks of the proper thickness will increase the filtration and reduce harmful secondary radiation; proper collimation will restrict the size of the primary beam; replacing the closed plastic cone with an open-ended PID (especially one with a scatter guard or lead-lining) further reduces secondary radiation; and replacing the mechanical timer with an electronic one will permit shorter exposure times. These modifications can be made at a modest expense and improve both safety and the diagnostic quality of the radiograph.

structural modifications

In many states it is required that dental rooms containing x-ray machines be provided with primary barriers (see definitions on page 60) at all areas struck by the useful beam, that protective barriers be provided between the x-ray rooms and near by operatories or hallways, and that each installation be provided with a protective barrier for the operator or be so arranged that he can stand at least six feet from the patient and away from the useful beam of radiation.

When these conditions cannot be met by relocating the x-ray machines or equipment in adjacent operatories, structural modifications must be made. In many cases structural materials of ordinary walls will suffice as a protective barrier without additional special shielding material. A wall made of two thicknesses of 5/8-inch gypsum board (1¼-inch total) can be assumed to provide minimum protection from scattered radiation only if the following conditions are met:

(1) The occupiable areas protected by the wall are at least six feet from the dental x-ray chair, (2) the x-ray operator is careful not to aim the primary x-ray beam at persons in areas adjacent to the x-ray room, and (3) the use of the x-ray equipment does not exceed 60 seconds/week of "on time" at 90 kVp or 100 seconds/week of "on time" at 65 kVp.

The average dental installation can usually meet the above conditions by proper layout and planning, and gypsum board or plastered walls will then provide adequate protection. For example, the primary beam can be directed toward an outside wall or into an unoccupied area. When these conditions cannot be met, as when two x-ray chairs are side by side, or when a receptionist sits immediately adjacent to the wall receiving the primary beam, additional structural shielding in the form of lead sheathing with a thickness of 1/32 inch is needed. When properly located, such lead shielding is almost always adequate in the dental office. The thickness and locations of these barriers should be determined by an individual qualified in x-ray shielding design.

In addition to this, darkroom modifications to prevent light leaks and the use of better processing equipment and chemicals—coupled with improved, standardized exposure and processing techniques— increase radiation safety and produce better radiographs.

radiation monitoring

The only way to make sure that x-ray equipment is not emitting too much radiation and people are not receiving more than the maximum permissible accumulated dose is to use monitoring devices. In radiography, *monitoring* is defined as "periodic or continuing measurement to determine the dose rate in a given area or the dose received by a person."

Radiation has four qualities that make accurate measurements possible: it affects photographic emulsions, produces ionization in air, produces a rise in temperature, and causes certain salts to fluoresce. All measuring devices make use of one of these qualities.

Area monitoring involves making an on-site survey to measure the output of the dental x-ray unit, to check for possible radiation leakage, and danger areas in the room (hot spots), and to determine if any radiation is passing through walls. Special equipment is needed to detect the exact amount of ionizing radiation at any given spot. Numerous firms specialize in monitoring. In some regions this service may be performed at the dentist's request by qualified state personnel.

Personnel monitoring requires office staff members to wear a device that measures how much radiation they are receiving. Monitoring devices vary in cost and effectiveness. Some merely indicate that radiation has been received; others show the amount, and still others measure the amount and type of radiation. In hospitals, industrial plants, and some dental offices, everyone working around radiation is required to wear a monitoring device at all times while on duty. The film badge and ionizing chambers are sufficiently accurate and economical to be worn in the dental offices. More and more dentists are providing monitoring devices and services for themselves and their employees. Pending legislation may soon make this mandatory in several states.

monitoring devices

The major problem with radiation measurements is that what we actually measure is the effect of radiation on photographic emulsion, on gas or air, and on certain crystals of fluorescent salts, rather than making a direct measurement of radiation itself; and for this we need monitoring devices.

The more complex devices, such as the Geiger counter and the scintillation counter, are not practical in the dental office and are included here only for the sake of completeness.

The Geiger counter contains a needle-like electrode inside a hollow metallic cylinder that is filled with gas which sets up a current in an electric field when it is ionized by radiation. The scintillation counter contains a photoelectric cell which helps to measure the flashes of visible light emitted when the radiation that bombards certain salt crystals within the instrument causes them to fluoresce.

Our major interest is in the personnel monitoring devices. The forerunner of these devices used in the dental office was an unexposed film to which a paper clip was attached. One wore it in a pocket with the clip and the exposure side of the film facing toward the outside. The film was developed at intervals ranging from a month to three months. Although extremely simple and economical, the shortcoming was that this home-made film badge showed only that radiation had been received and failed to record the amount of radiation.

A more sophisticated device is the pocket dosimeter, also called an ionization chamber. The dosimeter resembles a fountain pen and attaches to a garment with a clip. The dosimeter contains an ion chamber, a small sealed container of air designed so that the air can be ionized. The dosimeter can only be read when it is inserted into

Fig. 6–5   Film badge. (From *Answers to Your Questions About Radiation Monitoring*. Des Plaines, Illinois: Nuclear-Chicago Co. Courtesy of Nuclear-Chicago Co., A subsidiary of G. D. Searle & Co.)

a more complex piece of equipment called a charger-reader. When the ionized air is exposed to radiation, changes within the ion chamber can be measured through the movements of a spring electroscope when the dosimeter is inserted in the charger-reader. Some of the dosimeters are calibrated so that readings from 0 to 0.5 R can be observed. Dosimeters are very useful in installations with a high-work load because they can be recharged every morning and read at the end of the day; their disadvantage is that no permanent record of radiation is made.

A still more effective device is the modern film badge, a descendant of the paper clip device. A few firms provide a film badge service on a subscription basis. The cost is modest and decreases with the number of persons using it. Each subscriber is supplied with a badge loaded with a radiosensitive film. The plastic or metal holder is lined with various thicknesses of filters of different materials which make it possible to measure the types of radiation received while the film is in the badge (Fig. 6–5).

The badge is simple to load and has no dials to set or read. The film packet is simply removed at stated intervals and replaced with a new one. The exposed packet is mailed to a firm either weekly, bi-weekly, or monthly. Specialized equipment processes the film, measuring not only the amount but also the type of radiation. Each film is dated and marked with the subscriber's identifying number. A written report provides a clear and permanent record that shows the dose received while the film was worn, the accumulated dose for a 13-week period, and the total radiation accumulated during the year. In addition to providing early warning of overexposure to radiation, the service provides a permanent record. Subscribing to a film badge service is good insurance for dentists, because the courts recognize the films and records as evidence in a defense against damage claims.

bibliography

Answers to Your Questions About Radiation Monitoring, Des Plaines, Ill.: Nuclear-Chicago Corporation, 1968.

Kinsman, Simon, and Alcox, Ray W. *Radiation Hygiene in Dental Radiography,* Sacramento: State of California, Department of Public Health, Bureau of Radiological Health, 1970.

National Council on Radiation Protection and Measurements, NCRP Report No. 39, *Basic Radiation Protection Criteria,* Washington, D.C.: NCRP, 1971.

National Council on Radiation Protection and Measurements, NCRP Report No. 35, *Dental X-Ray Protection,* Washington, D.C.: NCRP, 1970.

O'Brien, Richard C. *Dental Radiography,* 2d ed. Philadelphia: W. B. Saunders Co., 1972.

Peterson, Shailer. *Clinical Dental Hygiene,* 3d ed. St. Louis: The C. V. Mosby Co., 1968.

Radiation Protection in Dental Practice, Sacramento: State of California, Department of Public Health, Bureau of Radiological Health, 1968.

Richardson, Richard E., and Barton, Roger E. *The Dental Assistant,* 4th ed. New York: McGraw-Hill Book Co., 1970.

Schwarzrock, Shirley Pratt, and Jensen, James R. *Effective Dental Assisting,* 4th ed. Dubuque, Iowa: William C. Brown Co., 1973.

Wainwright, William Ward. *Dental Radiology,* New York: McGraw-Hill Book Co., 1965.

Wilkins, Esther M. *Clinical Practice of the Dental Hygienist,* 3d ed. Philadelphia: Lea & Febiger, 1971.

Wuehrmann, Arthur H., and Manson-Hing, Lincoln R. *Dental Radiology,* 2d ed. St. Louis: The C. V. Mosby Co., 1969.

7

dental x-ray films

composition of dental x-ray films

Dental x-ray films are very similar to those used in photography;
in fact, the first dental radiograph was made on a photographic plate
a few weeks after Roentgen announced the discovery of the x-ray.
Dr. Otto Walkoff inserted an ordinary glass photographic plate, protected against light and moisture by an inner wrapping of black paper
and an outer wrapping of rubber dam, into his mouth and exposed it.
Although film emulsions and film packaging have undergone many
changes since that time, the fundamentals have not. The films used
in dental radiography are photographic films that have been especially
adapted in size, emulsion, film speed, and packaging to dental uses.

Most films used in dental radiography have a thin, flexible, clear
or blue-tinted polyester base. This base is about 0.008-inch thick—
the thickness deemed necessary for proper manipulation—and is
covered with a photographic emulsion on both sides (one side on
older films). This emulsion is composed of gelatin in which crystals
of silver halide salts are suspended. Halides are compounds of a
halogen (fluorine, chlorine, bromine, or iodine) with another element—
in photography, silver. Silver is most frequently combined with bromine in dental films.

This emulsion is sensitive to light, radiation, and bending. Great
care must be taken not to expose the film accidentally to radiation
or light. Minor bending can crack the surface of the emulsion and
major bending may loosen the protective wrapping and let in moisture or light.

During radiation, the emulsion covering the film base receives and
stores energy. This energy is the basis for the film's *latent image*,

which does not become visible until the film has been immersed in a sequence of chemicals at a given temperature for a given time. Film processing will be explained in Chapter 8.

film covering and packaging

The film manufacturer cuts the films to the sizes required in dentistry. Smaller films suitable for intraoral (inside the mouth) radiography are made into what is called a film packet. Larger films used in extraoral (outside the mouth) radiography are packed differently.

All intraoral film packets, regardless of manufacturer, are assembled similarly. The film is first surrounded by a black, light-proof paper; next, a thin sheet of lead foil is placed on the side of the film that will be away from the radiation source; an outer wrapping of moisture-resistant paper completes the assembly. The purpose of the lead foil backing is to absorb scattered radiation from striking the film emulsion from the back side of the film (the side away from the tube), thus fogging the film. A small tab for opening the film is located on the side away from the tube. To open it, one lifts the edge of the flap and pulls it back gently.

In most dental offices the film packet is referred to simply as the film. Each film (packet) has two sides—a *tube side* that faces the tube and a *back side* away from the source of radiation. The tube side is covered with white paper that is either smooth or slightly pebbly to prevent slippage. It also has a small embossed identifying dot near one of the corners. In intraoral radiography the tube side of the film faces the teeth to be x-rayed.

The back side containing the tab is smooth. Depending on the manufacturer, the entire back may be white or the tab portion may be colored. The following information is printed on the back side—manufacturer's name, film speed, the number of films in the packet (one or two), a circle or mark indicating the location of the identifying dot, and the legend "opposite side toward tube."

Most packets contains one film, but two-film packets are available. When a packet containing two x-ray films is exposed, duplicate radiographs result. This is useful whenever a radiograph is to be sent to another practitioner to whom the patient is referred (the other radiograph remains a part of the patient's permanent record), or a radiograph is needed for legal evidence.

Depending on the size, intraoral films are packaged 10, 25, 50, 144, or 150 to a box, the most popular being the 144 and 150 film packages. A layer of lead foil surrounds the films inside the box to protect them from damage by stray radiation or chemical fumes during storage.

film emulsion speeds (sensitivity)

The two main factors that determine film speed are the grain size of the silver halide crystals in the emulsion and whether one or both sides of the film base are coated. The slow films have the small grain size and only one coated side. Use of slow film is decreasing so much that many manufacturers have stopped making it.

Image definition (sharpness) is more distinct when grains are small. The large grains used in the earliest high-speed films resulted in a "graininess" that made the radiographs difficult to interpret. Improvements in manufacturing have made image definition almost as good on fast as on slow film. Film speeds (and image definition) are constantly improving.

The use of high-speed film has contributed more to radiation safety than any other single factor. Under ideal operating conditions, exposure can be reduced to a tiny fraction of what used to be considered necessary. Effective use of high-speed film is not practical unless the x-ray machine is equipped with an electronic timer and can be operated in the higher voltage ranges. Most modern offices have such machines.

Film names like "hyper," "super," "extra," and "ultra," tell little or nothing about the actual film speed. The standards for film speeds have been outlined by the Council on Research of the American Dental Association. Dental films are given ASA (speed) ratings from A for the slowest through F for the fastest. Most films used today are rated B, C, or D. The slow group B films are referred to as *regular,* the faster C films as *intermediate*, and the still faster D films as *fast* or *extra fast*. Although researchers are working with even faster speed films, the D speed film is the fastest one available at present and the one that is recommended.

types of dental x-ray films

The films used in dental radiography are classified according to use. The two main categories are *intraoral* films, designed principally for use inside the mouth, and *extraoral* films, to be used outside the mouth. However, an intraoral may be used to make an extraoral exposure. One may use any film whenever it can bring about the desired result.

X-ray machines taking *panoramic* films (in which all the teeth are shown on a single exposure) are becoming more common. At present, however, at least 95 percent of all radiographs are intraoral, including only the teeth and the tissues immediately surrounding them. Extraoral films are generally used to examine larger areas and to provide the dentist with supplemental information. Occasionally, as in the case of accidents or fractures, or for special situations, extraoral films may be used alone.

intraoral films

Three types of intraoral films, each named after its most common use, are: the *periapical,* the *interproximal* (bitewing), and the *occlusal* (Fig. 7-1).

Periapical films are used to make a detailed examination of the entire tooth, the periodontal membrane, and the surrounding bone tissues. Five sizes are manufactured (#00, #0, #1, #2, and #3)—the larger the number, the larger the film. Of these, #00 and #3 are used least frequently and not produced by all film manufacturers.

Numbers 00 and 0 films are especially designed for small children and thus are often called "pedo" (from Greek *paidos,* "child") or *pedodontic* films. Both the #1 and #2 films are most commonly used on larger children and adults. Use of the narrow #1 film is normally limited to exposing radiographs of the anterior teeth. Although it shows only two or three teeth, this film is ideal for areas where the mouth is narrow and curves a great deal. Its narrowness also makes it the best choice when film holders and the 16-inch target-film technique are used in the anterior areas of the mouth. The wider #2 film is generally referred to as the *standard* film. This film is used in at least 75 percent of all intraoral radiography. The extra-long #3 film, also called the *long bitewing* film, is rarely used as a periodontal film.

The *interproximal* (bitewing) films are used to examine the crowns of the teeth, the alveolar crests, and the surfaces of the teeth that touch each other. The exposures made with these films show the coronal portions of both the maxillary (upper) and mandibular (lower) teeth on the same film. They are particularly valuable when the dentist is trying to determine the extent of proximal caries between the teeth.

All interproximal films are available in the same sizes as the periapical films and have the same film numbers (refer to Fig. 7-1). The chief difference is that each film has a flap or tab attached to it on which the patient must bite to hold it in place between the occlusal surfaces of the maxillary and mandibular teeth. These films may be purchased with tabs. A periapical film can be converted to an interproximal film by being slipped into a commercially made cardboard

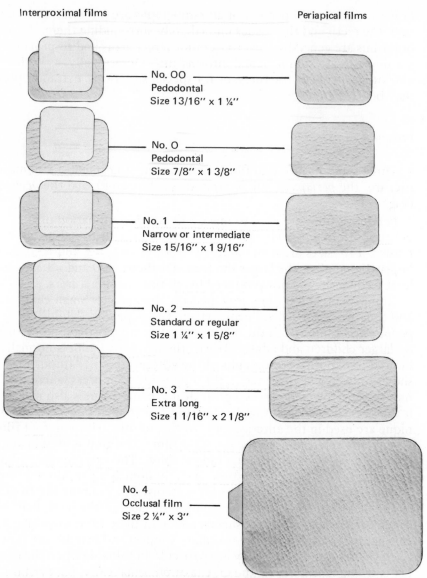

Interproximal films   Periapical films

No. OO
Pedodontal
Size 13/16" x 1 ¼"

No. O
Pedodontal
Size 7/8" x 1 3/8"

No. 1
Narrow or intermediate
Size 15/16" x 1 9/16"

No. 2
Standard or regular
Size 1 ¼" x 1 5/8"

No. 3
Extra long
Size 1 1/16" x 2 1/8"

No. 4
Occlusal film
Size 2 ¼" x 3"

Fig. 7-1 With the exception of the large occlusal films that are used occlusally
or extraorally on occasions, all intraoral films are available in two forms: Plain for
periapical use or with an attached bite tab for interproximal (bitewing) use.
(Courtesy of Rinn Corporation, Dental X-Ray Division.)

film loop (Fig. 7–2), or having a piece of scotch tape wrapped around
it to form a tab.

The *occlusal* films (#4) are the largest of the intraoral films. The
patient normally holds them in position by biting directly on them.

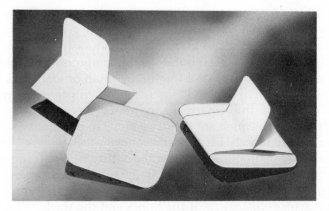

Fig. 7-2 Bite loops for interproximal (bitewing) films. Bite loops offer an easy way to convert film from periapical to interproximal use. The loop is spread open and the desired film is centered into the loop. The plain side of the film must face toward the bite tab and the source of radiation. Bite loops are available in various sizes. (Courtesy of Rinn Corporation, Dental X-Ray Division.)

These films are ideal for making a rapid survey of a large area of the maxilla, mandible, and floor of the mouth. They can reveal gross pathological lesions, root fragments, bone and tooth fractures, and impacted or supernumerary teeth and many other conditions. Occlusal films may be used to make a rapid survey of an edentulous (without teeth) mouth or of the mouth of a child who is afraid to hold one of the smaller periapical films tightly against the teeth.

Occlusal films are often used extraorally for radiographs of the third molar areas when it is not practical to place a film far back in the mouth or when the patient's face is swollen and opening the mouth is difficult. This versatile film has many other uses which will be considered later in the text. Although only the #4 film is called the occlusal film, periapical films of any size can be used to make occlusal exposures.

extraoral films

The larger extraoral films are generally packaged 25, 50, or 100 to a box. With the exception of films sold in "Ready-Pack" envelopes, films are sandwiched between two pieces of protective paper and the entire group is wrapped in lead foil for protection. Because these films are designed for extraoral use, they require neither individual lead backings or moistureproof wrappings. The films vary in size depending on what area is to be radiographed. The most common sizes are 5 in. by 7 in., used mainly for lateral views of the jaw, 8 in. by 10 in., used for profiles and posteronanterior views, and 5 in. or

6 in. by 12 in., for panoramic radiographs of the entire dentition.

The large extraoral films are used to examine gross structures such as the skull, the maxilla and mandible in relationship to each other, or specific areas of the facial bones or the temporomandibular joint. They can show the extent of a fracture, growth or malignancy and can be used to study jaw development, tooth eruption, or any of a long list of normal and abnormal conditions. Except for the panoramic radiographs, which are rapidly gaining in popularity, extraoral films are not frequently used by the general practitioners. Their major users are orthodontists, prosthodontists, and oral surgeons.

Orthodontists use facial profile radiographs (*cephalometric—*meaning "measuring the head") periodically to record, measure, and compare changes in growth of the bones and the teeth.

The prosthodontists use facial profile radiographs to record the contour of the lips and face and the relationship of the teeth before removal. This helps them to construct prosthetic appliances that look natural.

Oral surgeons use extraoral radiographs extensively to determine the location and extent of fractures and to locate imbedded teeth, abnormalities, malignancies, and injuries to the temporomandibular joint.

Two types of extraoral films are available—non-screen and screen films. Each of these is coated with emulsion on both sides; however, the thickness of the emulsion and its sensitivity to radiation and light vary.

Non-screen film is designed for use in a cardboard exposure holder. Because the x-rays must penetrate more tissues in extraoral exposures, the emulsion has to be thicker than that used in intraoral films; otherwise the exposure times would be too long. The emulsion of non-screen film is more sensitive to the x-rays than it is to blue or violet lights that are produced when x-rays strike an intensifying screen and cause its crystals to glow or fluoresce.

Screen film, as the name suggests, is designed to be used in a holder lined with *intensifying screens.* Such a holder is called a cassette. The emulsion of screen film is more sensitive to the blue and violet lights, emitted when the x-rays strike the crystals of the intensifying screens that line the cassette, causing a fluorescent light to act on the exposed film within the cassette, than they are to the x-rays themselves. The term intensifying screens is used because the fluorescent action intensifies the energy produced within the cassette and reduces the required exposure time and permits the use of a thinner emulsion than with non-screen film.

The advantage of non-screen film is that it can be used in a light-weight exposure holder. It produces satisfactory radiographs in areas such as the lateral jaw, where a minimum of tissue must be penetrated. Its disadvantage is that it requires an exposure time that is too long in areas of great density, where the x-rays have to pass through the tissues of the entire head before they reach the film. Screen film must be used for such exposures.

Since all extraoral films, with the exception of the "Ready-Pack" films are wrapped only in an interleaving paper which protects them from contact with each other in the box that holds them, they must be loaded into the exposure holder or cassette under darkroom conditions to prevent damage by exposure to light.

exposure holders and cassettes

Both exposure holders and cassettes are available in sizes that correspond to the most frequently used extraoral films. In fact, an intraoral cassette large enough to hold the occlusal film is manufactured. This, however, is used seldom except by specialists. The cassettes, being of metal construction, are heavier and more difficult for the patients to hold. Special devices to position and hold these cassettes are required in several techniques.

Exposure holders consist of two pieces of cardboard that are hinged on one end and have a metal clasp on the other end to lock the holder after the film is inserted. An envelope, whose flaps can be opened or closed, is visible when the holder is open. This envelope serves to contain the non-screen film and protect it from visible light rays. The interleaving paper around the film is left in place since it does not interfere with the passage of the x-rays and serves as an additional protection against light in the flimsily constructed holder.

In dental radiography the source of radiation is always from the direction opposite to the side of the face against which the film is placed. The tube side of the holder has the words "tube side" printed on it and is positioned in contact with the patient's face or head. The back side of the holder contains a lead backing to help absorb some of the exit radiation and to protect the patient's hand while he steadies the holder during the exposure.

Cassettes are rigid holders (usually aluminum) that consist of a lid and a base. The lid (tube side) consists of a narrow metal frame that surrounds the thin plastic layer that forms the *face* of the cassette. Plastic is used because it offers only slight resistance to the passage of x-rays. The base (back side) is made of solid metal that absorbs much

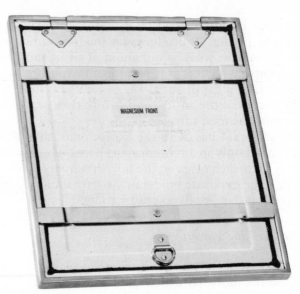

Fig. 7-3 View of the back of a cassette. The front contacts the skin of the patient and faces toward the source of radiation. The film is placed between the intensifying screens. The hinge and clamps are for opening and closing the cassette. The film must be loaded or unloaded in the darkroom with special subdued light and the clamps on the cassette must be absolutely tight to prevent light leakage. (Courtesy of General Electric, Medical Systems Division.)

of the exit radiation. Although extraoral cassettes can be used without intensifying screens (in which case they function similarly to an exposure holder, but are of sturdier construction), the majority contain a built-in intensifying screen in both the lid and the base. Hinges fasten the lid to the base and permit easy opening and closing. One or two clamps on the back of the base make it possible to close the cassette tightly (Fig. 7-3).

Strong spring-type clamps are used to close the cassette because the action of the intensifying screens is most effective when the film is tightly pressed against the screens. The protective paper surrounding the film must be removed when the screen film is placed in the cassette; otherwise the blue or purple light rays emanating from the screens could not reach the film surface.

An *intensifying screen* is a smooth cardboard or plastic sheet coated with minute fluorescent crystals mixed into a suitable binding medium. It produces the desired image in a shorter exposure time than is possible with non-screen film in a cardboard exposure holder. It is based on the principle that crystals of certain salts—in this case, calcium tungstate or barium lead sulfate—will fluoresce and emit energy in the form of blue, violet, or ultraviolet light when they

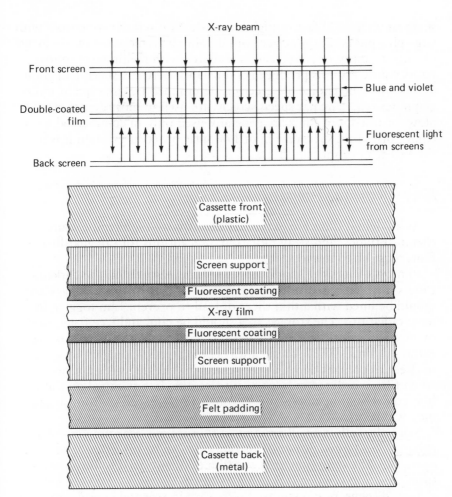

Fig. 7–4 Cross-section of cassette and diagram showing the cumulative effect of x-ray and fluorescent light on the film. (From Ennis, Leroy M. et al, *Dental Roentgenology*. Philadelphia: Lea & Febiger, 1967.)

absorb x-rays. Each of these fluorescent crystals, also called *phosphors*, gives off blue to ultraviolet radiations that vary in intensity according to the x-rays in that part of the image. As already observed, screen film is more sensitive to this type light than to radiation. When the film is sandwiched tightly between two intensifying screens, the wasted heat that accompanies x-rays, along with the x-rays themselves, cause the crystals on the screens to fluoresce and return the emitted light to the emulsion to intensify the radiographic image (Fig. 7–4).

Intensifying screens are available in three speeds: (1) Slow or high-definition screens are coated with small phosphors and produce the sharpest image; (2) fast or high-intensification screens are coated with large phosphors that produce considerably less sharpness of the image; (3) intermediary or *par* screens are coated with medium-size phosphors whose crystals produce good balance between speed and good definition. The choice of screens is determined by the type of radiograph desired. The par speed screens are used in most dental offices. Slow- or fast-speed films are generally used only in commercial x-ray laboratories that specialize in orthodontic procedures when it is desired to achieve special effects.

film protection and storage

As all dental films are extremely sensitive to high temperatures, chemical fumes, and stray radiation, precautions for safeguarding films must be followed.

In most offices the supply of x-ray films is stored in the darkroom. Unless it is quite far from the nearest x-ray machine, the storage area should be lined with a thin sheet of lead to prevent film fogging by stray radiation. The storage area should be cool and free from humidity or chemical vapors. Particular care must be taken when storing extraoral films. They should always be stored standing up, not stacked, to prevent damaging or scratching the delicate emulsion. When film is ordered in large quantities, the date stamped on the film box should be noted and the older films placed in front so that they will be used first.

Normally only a small amount of film is kept near the x-ray machine. A lead-lined dispenser or film safe can be placed near the operator. The only time that the film does not need to be protected from radiation is when it is being exposed.

Film dispensers and storage boxes vary in size and complexity. The simplest storage box is a lead-lined container with a removable lead-lined lid. Slightly more complex is a wall-mounted radiation-resistant container. Films are loaded from the top and stacked vertically into a film chute that holds about 150 single or double film packets. A dispensing mechanism delivers one film out of the slot at the bottom of the dispenser each time a plunger is pressed and released. This type dispenser is available with chutes to fit the most commonly used films. A more complex dispenser is designed to handle #0, #1, and #2 films simultaneously (Fig. 7–5). It contains an additional storage area for interproximal and occlusal film.

A small lead-lined safe or receptacle is used to protect exposed film from additional exposure while other radiographs are being made on the same patient. Such receptacles usually hold a maximum

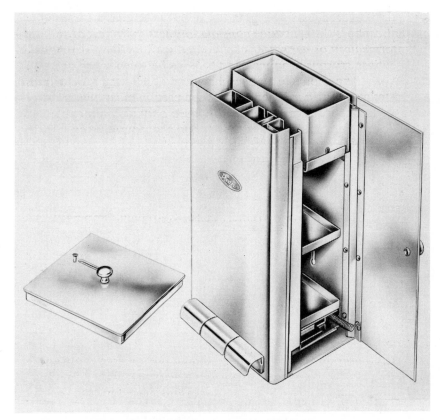

Fig. 7-5 Film dispenser with chutes and space for various sizes of intraoral films. (Courtesy of Rinn Corporation, Dental X-Ray Division.)

of 24 to 30 films. Immediately after exposure, the used film is carefully wiped or blotted to remove saliva and is dropped into the receptacle through a slot in its top. After all exposures are completed, films should be removed immediately and taken to the darkroom for processing.

film requirements

There is no hard and fast rule for the number of films required to make a full-mouth exposure. One rule is to use the largest films that can be placed effectively and tolerated by the patient. This will enable the operator to complete the survey with a minimum of exposures. However, the operator should remember that because of the curvature of the mouth, normally only two or three teeth—and occasionally only one tooth—can be viewed on any single film without distortion. Normally, one places the films in the mouth so that each overlaps the next, to show some of the same structures.

A minimum of 14 periapical films are required—more if the narrow #1 films are used in the anterior regions—for a routine full-mouth survey of an adult patient with all his teeth. Such a survey includes a minimum of 2 interproximal films. The ideal full-mouth series consists of 18 to 21 films.

When a routine examination of an edentulous mouth is made, two occlusal films are used—one for the maxilla and one for the mandible. Periapical films are used to supplement the molar regions and any other area that the dentist wants to look at.

For a child, the type of film varies with his age, size, and emotional stability. Generally such examinations include two interproximal films and at least ten #00 or #0 periapical films.

Conditions may require more or less film for any examination. For example, development of routine x-rays may reveal unusual or unexpected conditions that make more exposures necessary. The dentist, the operator, or both determine the number and type of films to be used and the duration of the exposures.

bibliography

Ennis, Leroy M., Berry, Harrison M., and Phillips, James E. *Dental Roentgenology*, 6th ed. Philadelphia: Lea & Febiger, 1967.

O'Brien, Richard C. *Dental Radiography*, 2d ed. Philadelphia: W. B. Saunders Co., 1972.

Peterson, Shailer. *Clinical Dental Hygiene,* 3d ed. St. Louis: The C. V. Mosby Co., 1968.

Richardson, Richard E., and Barton, Roger E. *The Dental Assistant*, 4th ed. New York: McGraw-Hill Book Co., 1970.

Schwarzrock, Shirley Pratt, and Jensen, James R. *Effective Dental Assisting*, 4th ed. Dubuque, Iowa: William C. Brown Co., 1973.

Wainwright, William Ward. *Dental Radiology*, New York: McGraw-Hill Book Co., 1965.

Wilkins, Esther M. *Clinical Practice of the Dental Hygienist*, 3d ed. Philadelphia: Lea & Febiger, 1971.

Wuehrmann, Arthur M., and Manson-Hing, Lincoln R. *Dental Radiology*, 2d ed. St. Louis: The C. V. Mosby Co., 1969.

X-Rays in Dentistry, Rochester, N.Y.: Eastman Kodak Co., 1972.

8

dental

x-ray film processing

fundamentals of film processing

Photography and radiography are similar both in the films they use
and in techniques used to process them. Both photographic and radiographic films are extremely sensitive to light and can be processed
only in a properly equipped darkroom or special processing units.
Processing transforms the latent image, which is produced when the
energy of the x-ray photons is absorbed by the silver halide crystals
in the emulsion (energy of the light rays in the case of photographic
film), into a visible, stable image by means of chemicals.

The processing of photographic and radiographic film is based on
five simple facts: (1) Compounds of silver and halogens are sensitive
to light and x-radiation; (2) a photographic or radiographic film consists of a polyester base covered with emulsion of silver halide grains
(crystals) suspended in a solution of gelatin; (3) the function of the
gelatin is to keep the silver halide grains evenly suspended over the
base; (4) the gelatin will not dissolve in cold water but it swells, thus
exposing the silver halide grains to the chemicals in the developing
solution; and (5) the gelatin shrinks as it dries, leaving a smooth surface that becomes the negative or radiograph.

During the chemical processing a selective reduction of the exposed
silver halide grains takes place. Selective reduction means that the
non-metallic elements—the halides—are removed. Only the exposed
silver remains (Fig. 8–1).

During processing the halides on the film are reduced when immersed in the *developer* for a predetermined interval (a time-temperature cycle is generally used). The bromide in the exposed halides is

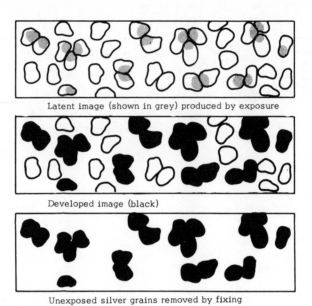

Latent image (shown in grey) produced by exposure

Developed image (black)

Unexposed silver grains removed by fixing

Fig. 8-1 On exposure to radiation or light, a latent image is formed that is made visible through the developing procedure. (From Baker, Benjamin R., and Strickland, William D. *Dental Assisting*, Course VII, Clinical Application, 2d ed. Chapel Hill, N.C.: University of North Carolina Press, 1971.)

removed by the chemicals of the developer and the metallic silver, which turns black, remains. The unexposed halide grains (in film areas opposite metallic or dense structures that adsorb and prevent the passage of x-ray photons) are unaffected at this time. After brief rinsing to remove any developer remaining on the film, the film is immersed in the *fixer* for approximately double the developing time. The unexposed halides are removed during this interval, leaving behind only the metallic silver which is not disturbed by the chemicals of the fixer solution. Thus, the images on the film are made up of microscopic grains of black metallic silver. The amount of silver deposited will vary with the thickness of the tissues penetrated. Where only soft tissues were between the source of the radiation and the emulsion, the film will be black. It will be white where passage of x-rays was blocked by metal fillings or restorations.

As we have already seen in Chapter 4, the amount of light transmitted through the film varies according to the thickness of tissues penetrated by the radiation and accounts for the shades of black, gray, and white. Dark areas are spoken of as radiolucent and light ones as radiopaque. After the film is completely fixed, it is washed for a minimum of twenty minutes to remove any remaining traces of the chemicals of the fixer and then allowed to dry.

In radiography, as in photography, both exposure and processing must be standardized for good results. For example, dried chemicals, dust, or dirt on the workbench can spoil what would otherwise have been an excellent radiograph. Failure to regulate the temperature of the water and the solutions in the processing tanks can have dire consequences, as the emulsion can melt in warm water. High-speed films are extremely sensitive to variations in light, temperature, and processing chemicals—more so than are slow or intermediate films. The price of obtaining a good radiograph is meticulous attention to detail.

darkroom and equipment

Until recently, a darkroom was absolutely necessary for processing films. Now automatic processing machines may be used in normal light, but a darkroom will probably still be required to load and un-load exposure holders or cassettes, to process certain films, and just to be there in case the automatic processing equipment breaks down.

In some offices the darkroom is a large, well-equipped, convenient room; in others it is just an afterthought. Certainly, the size and equipment of the darkroom will contribute little to the production of good radiographs if exposure or processing is poor, but a well-equipped room makes good, standardized processing much easier. As with all things, some darkroom equipment is essential and some is merely nice to have.

However, cleanliness and orderliness are essential. Since the films are handled in almost complete darkness, usually with just a very dim safelight, all needed materials must be within easy reach and the person doing the processing must know where each item is kept. The workbench must be absolutely free from water, dust, chemicals, or any other substance that can come in contact with unwrapped film. Particular care must be taken not to splash chemical solutions or water on the bench when moving films from one insert of the developing tank to the other. A messy darkroom is not only unpleasant to work in but can stain and damage clothes. More seriously, dirty darkrooms can produce worthless radiographs.

The ideal darkroom is the result of good planning. It is large enough to meet the requirements of the office, is arranged with ample work space, is equipped with the correct types of light, is well ventilated, and has adequate storage space for films and radiographic supplies. The darkroom should be an adequate distance from the nearest x-ray machine and should not be used as a general storage area, especially not for materials that produce dust or give off chemical fumes.

The following items are absolutely essential in the darkroom: (1) a normal electric light for use when the films are not being processed, (2) a darkroom safelight, (3) a processing tank, (4) a utility sink, (5) racks for film hangers for holding and drying the radiographs, (6) brushes to clean the tank, (7) paddles to stir the solution, (8) drip pans to place under wet hangers, (9) storage racks for the film hangers, (10) a timer, (11) two thermometers, and (12) a wastebasket or waste disposal chute. Not essential but nice to have are: (1) an electric fan or film dryer, (2) additional safelights—preferably with foot control switches, (3) a built-in view box or illuminator, (4) controls for regulating the temperature of the water entering the processing tank, (5) a safety "in-use" light, and (6) ample storage facilities for films and radiographic supplies.

darkroom illumination

Although most darkrooms are painted black, they need not be as long as the darkroom is completely sealed to white light. Felt strips may have to be installed around the door or any other area where a light leak is discovered. Fluorescent overhead light should not be used because of its afterglow.

Two types of safelights may be used in the darkroom. The first is the filtered Wratten 6B series—a red bulb that gives off a minimum of light and can be used for processing any type of dental film. A 7-1/2 watt bulb is used when the light is within 3 feet above the work area; a larger 15 watt is used for distances over 6 feet (Fig. 8-2). The other type of safelight provides considerably more illumination and can be used only with some films. This type of light cannot be used when loading or unloading exposure holders and cassettes or when processing extraoral films. The manufacturer indicates in bold faced type on the outside of the box containing the films whether safelights, which give off added light, may be used.

Any light, whether white or safelight, has the capacity to fog or darken the radiograph. To find out if your light is really safe, unwrap a film that has been exposed under normal conditions and place it on the workbench. Center a coin on the film and leave it exposed to the glow of the safelight for 30 minutes before developing it. If the processed film shows any sign of a circle where the coin was placed, the light given off by the safelight is excessive.

Some darkrooms are equipped with wall-type view boxes or illuminators. These give off considerable light, and care must be taken not to unwrap films or leave the cover of the processing tank off when these are turned on. If the darkroom can be locked, this should be

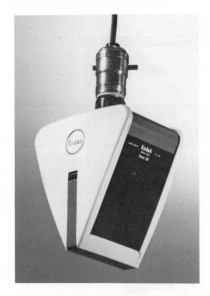

Fig. 8-2 The Kodak two-way safelight. This safelight can be supplied with a 15-watt bulb and a Kodak safelight filter, Type ML-2, or with a 7½-watt incandescent lamp and Kodak safelight filter, Wratten 6B series. It can be used when developing any dental x-ray films. Other types are available that give off more light. Their use, however, is restricted to films that can tolerate more light. (Courtesy of The Eastman Kodak Company.)

done before processing is started to prevent anyone from entering and inadvertently spoiling the films through exposure to light; otherwise, the "in-use" light must be turned on.

processing tanks

Several types and sizes of processing tanks are available. Most used in dental offices are large enough to accept an 8 in. by 10 in. extraoral film. They hold one gallon of developer and one gallon of fixer in separate compartments, with a large central area in between for rinsing and washing the films (Fig. 8-3).

The processing tank may be made in one piece or with two removable inserts. It may be entirely of hard rubber, have a hard rubber core with stainless steel inserts, or be made entirely of stainless steel with welded and polished joints to prevent a reaction with the processing chemicals. Most tanks have removable inserts to facilitate cleaning, and a small hole at the bottom of the insert lets the solution drain into the central compartment when a small rubber plug is pulled out. The central section is connected to the water intake and to the drain. When in use, fresh water circulates constantly. An overflow pipe keeps the level of the water constant when the tank is full. Some tanks are equipped with a temperature control device that mixes the hot and cold water in the pipes to any desired temperatures. A close-fitting light-proof cover completes the tank assembly.

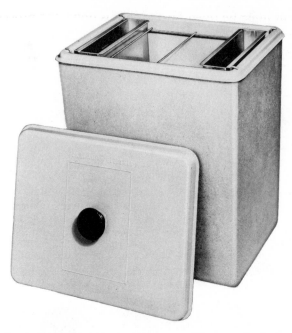

Fig. 8-3 Developing tank with removable inserts. The central compartment holds the rinse water. Generally, the insert on the left is filled with the developer solution and the insert of the right is filled with the fixer solution. (Courtesy of General Electric, Medical Systems Division.)

care of tanks and processing solutions

The operator should always wear a protective plastic or rubber apron when cleaning the tank or changing the solutions. The tank and its inserts should be scrubbed each time that the solutions are changed. A solution made up of 1.5 oz. commercial hydrochloric acid, a quart of cold water, and three quarts of warm water is sufficient to remove the deposits that frequently form on the walls of one-gallon inserts. To clean the processing tank, first pull the plug and drain the inserts, then thoroughly scrub all portions of tank, inserts, and cover. If the inserts appear to be coated, fill them with acid cleaning solution and let them soak for half an hour; then drain out the cleaning solution and rinse them with plenty of water. All parts of the tank, including the cover, should be wiped clean before the plugs are replaced and the inserts filled.

After the developer and the fixer are poured into the inserts until the level of the solutions reaches a mark on the side of the insert that indicates the full level (about one inch from the top), the central compartment must be filled. When that is done, the processing tank is ready for use. Most operators drain the central compartment at the end of each working day.

Whenever possible, the processing tank should remain covered to prevent oxidation, evaporation, and/or contamination of the processing solutions. The developer is especially subject to oxidation in the presence of air and loses some of its effectiveness. Oxidation is the union of a substance—in this case, the developer—with air. The cover should be removed only when adding solutions to the proper level, when checking the temperature of the developer or the water, and when inserting, removing, or changing the film hangers from one compartment or insert to another. The cover should be replaced immediately after any of these steps is completed.

Chemical contamination is an ever-present threat in film processing. Stirring paddles and thermometers must be cleaned after each use. Film hangers must be thoroughly rinsed to prevent chemicals from sticking to the handles before they are dried and ready for attaching the film. Care must be taken not to rotate the cover when it is removed, thereby causing a drop or two of condensed developer to fall into the fixer or vice versa. The operator can minimize this threat by labeling the inserts and the cover and by always refilling the inserts with the same solution that was originally placed in them and by making sure that the part of the cover over the developer is always placed there.

x-ray processing solutions

As already indicated, the chief processing chemicals are in the developer, which is slightly alkaline, and in the fixer, which is slightly acid. Both the developer and the fixer contain four constituents, each of which makes a specific contribution to the development or fixing process. The vehicle for mixing these ingredients is preferably distilled water; however, tap water is often used provided it is known to contain no interfering chemicals.

The main purpose of the developer is to reduce the exposed halide grains, loosening the exposed bromides and leaving the metallic silver on the film base in a specific arrangement depending on the thickness of the tissues or structures exposed or the mAs, kVp, or distances used. Four constituents are required to accomplish this: (1) a developing agent (also called a reducing agent), (2) a preservative, (3) an activator (also called an alkalizer), and (4) a restrainer.

The *developing agent* contains two chemicals—hydroquinone and elon. Although both chemicals are more active at higher than at lower temperatures, the hydroquinone becomes extremely active when the temperature of the solution is raised and is inactive at lower temperatures. The hydroquinone works slowly but steadily to build up density and contrast in the film, while the elon works fast but produces details slowly. Although these two chemicals affect the film contrast differently, the temperature of the developer affects the contrast shown on the radiograph. Thus, the higher the temperature, the less time is required to develop the film.

The *preservative*, sodium sulfite, protects the developing agents by slowing down the rapid oxidation rate of the developer.

The *activator*, sodium carbonate, provides the necessary alkaline medium required to accomplish reduction, and softens and swells the gelatin letting more of the exposed silver bromide grains come in contact with the developing agents.

The *restrainer*, potassium bromide, slows down the action of both development agents and inhibits the tendency of the solution to chemically fog the film.

The function of the fixer is to stop further development—thereby establishing the image permanently on the film—to remove the unexposed silver bromide grains (those that were not exposed to x-rays), and to harden the emulsion. Four constituents are required to accomplish this: (1) a fixing agent, (2) a preservative, (3) a hardening agent, and (4) an acidifier. The result of this process is a negative (radiographs are negatives while photographs are positives) that shows a graduation of light and dark corresponding to the layers of microscopic silver deposited.

The *fixing agent* is sodium thiosulfate, also known as "hypo" or hyposulfate of sodium. It removes all unexposed and any remaining undeveloped silver bromide grains from the emulsion.

The *preservative* is sodium sulfite (same chemical as used in developer). It slows down the rate of oxidation and prevents the deterioration of the hypo and the precipitation of sulfur.

The *hardening agent*, potassium alum, shrinks and hardens the emulsion. This hardening continues until the film is dry, thus protecting it from abrasion.

The *acidifier*, acetic acid, provides the acid medium required to neutralize the alkali of the developer and stop further development.

Two other chemicals are sometimes used in processing radiographs—a wetting agent and a cutting reducer. A *wetting agent* reduces the surface tension of the film. A teaspoon of wetting agent added to the developer will hasten even film development. Moreover, the fully processed film will dry much faster if, after being properly washed, it is immersed for one minute in a pan of water to which a few drops of wetting agent have been added.

A *cutting reducer* is a combination of potassium ferricyanide and fixer. It can be used in an emergency to lighten films that have been accidentally overexposed or overdeveloped. The use of a cutting reducer is indicated only when the film is too dark to diagnose and it is impossible or inadvisable to retake the film. Because much of the film density is lost when a reducer is used, this procedure should be attempted only as a last resort. The procedure varies slightly with the brand. Instructions should be checked carefully. The negative must be wet before reduction is started; if the film is already dry it must first be soaked in water for 10 minutes. Since the reducing action progresses very rapidly by removing successive layers of metallic silver, the negative must be closely watched. When enough reduction has taken place, the negative must be rinsed, fixed for 5 minutes, and washed for 20 minutes.

The chemicals used in development and fixation may be obtained in powder form, ready mixed in gallon jugs, or in liquid concentrate form. When used in powder form distilled water must be added and prolonged stirring is necessary to properly dissolve the crystals. The advantage of the powdered form is that solutions made from it are always fresh; the disadvantage is that it takes longer to mix. The advantage of the ready-mix is that it only needs to be opened and poured into the insert. The disadvantages are that the bottles are bulky, which may cause a storage problem, and the solution may not be as fresh. The concentrate form (Fig. 8–4) is used in most offices. It is easy to store, is fresh, and can be prepared in a few minutes. In many cities, regular tank cleaning and solution changing services are available.

The processing solutions should be changed every two or three weeks—more often if the traffic in radiographs is extremely heavy. Three things affect the useful life of the solution: the original quality or concentration of the solution, determined by how carefully the proportions are measured and how the solution is stirred; the freshness of the solution; and the number of films that are processed in it.

A small but significant amount of developer is lost daily through evaporation and by drops of developer adhering to the film surfaces and the film hanger as they are transferred to the rinse compartment. The loss in the fixer is smaller; actually some dilution takes place by rinse water clinging to the film and hanger when they are transferred to the fixer. Since some fixer is lost when the film hanger is subsequently removed, these factors about balance. The main loss of the fixer is from evaporation; the gradual dilution weakens the solution.

Opinions differ as to whether it is better to change the processing solutions more frequently or to replenish (raise the solution levels to the full mark by topping-off the tank inserts) them as needed. One

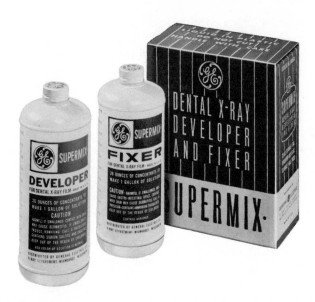

Fig. 8-4 Typical concentrate forms of developer and fixer. Each bottle is mixed with sufficient water to make 1 gallon of solution, which is the normal capacity of an insert. The solutions also may be made from dry materials or may be obtained in ready-mixed form. (Courtesy of General Electric, Medical Systems Division.)

of the first signs of developer exhaustion is light film with a thin image. Fixer exhaustion can be recognized when the film has not cleared in two minutes and still shows a milky coating. One satisfactory way to prolong the life of the solutions is to replenish them periodically. Some extra solution can be mixed and stored in tightly capped bottles to prevent oxidation until needed. Some operators make it a practice to top-off the inserts every morning. In addition to compensation for losses from evaporation and dripping off hangers, the addition of fresh chemicals helps to maintain the overall strength of the solutions. One hazard of permitting the solution levels to drop is that there may not be sufficient developer or fixer to cover all of the films attached to the uppermost clips of the film hanger. This may go unnoticed in the dim light of the darkroom and result in a partial image on the radiograph. This will not happen if the inserts are topped-off daily.

Sometimes technicians overexpose or overdevelop the film when the solutions become weak. They should not, because overexposure subjects everyone to more radiation than necessary. Overdevelopment is inaccurate and results in a loss of diagnostic film quality.

processing procedure

The completion of the radiograph involves preparation for processing, film processing, and final procedures. Each of these involve a number of steps.

The key to processing dental radiographs is adequate preparation. *Preparation* includes: (1) filling the rinse compartment with fresh circulating water, checking the solution levels, and stirring the developer and fixer thoroughly to prevent the heavier chemical from settling to the bottom; (2) determining the temperatures of the water and the developer; (3) checking one's hands and the workbench for cleanliness, selecting the proper film hangers, determining the optimum development time and setting the timer, laying out the film on the workbench, and identifying the films on the hanger; and (4) closing the darkroom door, turning off all lights except the selected safelight, unwrapping the film packets and securing them to the clips on the hanger. Some of these steps require further explanation.

Although films can be developed by the visual method, in which the films in the developer are removed several times and observed with the safelight to determine whether the images of the teeth can be clearly seen, this is not practical in dental radiography and does not standardize the technique. For this reason, the time-temperature method has been adopted by most operators. Directions on printed charts and manufacturer's directions will tell you how to follow it. Depending on the brand of film being used, a development time of either 4½ or 5 minutes is suggested when the temperatures of the developer and the water are at 68°F. Following the chart one can see how much more time is required if the water and the developer are colder and how much less if they are warmer. The water should be allowed to circulate in the tank long enough before the films are placed in it for processing to even the temperatures in all three compartments of the tank. Temperature variations of approximately 8 degrees from the ideal of 68°F. are acceptable, as long as the developing time is correspondingly reduced as the temperature increases and vice versa. Much lower temperatures make the chemical reaction sluggish, with poor results. With higher temperatures the danger of fogging the film increases; when the temperatures exceed 80 degrees, the gelatin in the emulsion begins to melt. A floating thermometer should be kept in both the developer insert and in the water compartment for frequent temperature reading (Fig. 8-5).

The selection of the proper film hanger and the identification of the film must also be considered. Decide what type and how many

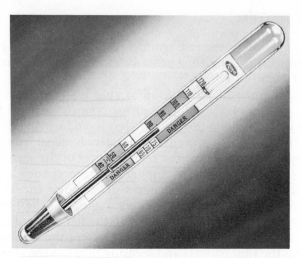

Fig. 8-5 Floating thermometer for use in the developer solution or water compartment. When using the time-temperature method, the ideal temperature ranges between 68° and 70°F. (Courtesy of Rinn Corporation, Dental X-Ray Division.)

films are to be processed and select the film hanger that will suit the task. Intraoral film hangers hold from 1 to 16 periapical or interproximal films (fewer occlusal films). Most have a white plastic identification tag near the handle on which the patient's name can be entered (Fig. 8-6). This tab can be erased and used again after the film is removed from it and positively identified on a mount or in an envelope. Extraoral films are best identified by fastening an identification plate to one of the lower corners of the face of the exposure holder or cassette. Special lettering sets are available. Minimum identification is the patient's name and the letters R (for right) and L (for left). These identifications become visible on the processed radiograph.

All radiographs to be processed must be identified in some manner; those that cannot be identified are completely worthless to the dentist. A good procedure is to enter the patient's name and the number of films exposed on him in a record book kept in the darkroom. This is particularly important in a busy office where the traffic in radiographs is heavy. At the end of the day it is virtually impossible to remember what films were exposed, and unless orderly records are kept, dangerous mixups, loss of time, and embarrassment can result.

Before processing can begin, the films must be removed from their protective wrappers or the cassette and fastened to the selected film hanger. There are four steps in preparing the intraoral film packet for processing: (1) Pull up and out on the film tab to tear open the

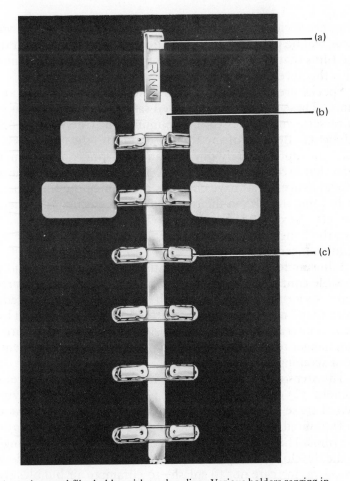

Fig. 8–6   An intraoral film holder with twelve clips. Various holders ranging in capacity from a single film to sixteen films are available. (a) Curved portion at top of holder rests on upper rim of tank insert when films are immersed. (b) White plastic identification tag on which the patient's name can be written in pencil and later erased. (c) Clamps with three point positive grip hold the film securely in place and parallel to the film base. (Courtesy of Rinn Corporation, Dental X-Ray Division.)

top of the packet; (2) pull on the tab until approximately half of the black paper is out of the packet; (3) hold the black paper away from the film and carefully remove the film from the packet, grasping the film by the edge so as not to smudge the surface of the film; and (4) clip the film to the hanger, testing each film to check whether it is securely held by the clip; failure to do this may cause the film to be lost at the bottom of the tank. Some film packets contain two films; however, only one film may be attached to each clip. If two films are accidentally fastened to the same clip, only the outside surfaces will be properly developed because the emulsion on the sides of the films that face each other will not come into sufficient contact with the developer and fixer.

Special precautions must be followed with the larger extraoral films. These can only be removed safely from the exposure holder or cassette and processed in minimum light (the Wratten 6B-type safelight). Because of the thicker emulsion, the non-screen films require an approximately one and one-half longer development time than that used for intraoral films. Extraoral films are placed in special hangers that have channels into which the film fits. Do this by holding the film in the right hand and grasping the hanger with the left. Next, guide the film into the channels until it is all the way into the hanger and the hinged retaining channel over the open end of the hanger can be closed.

Films undergoing processing must hang individually and out of possible contact with other films or with the side of the processing tank. As a rule, when a tank with one-gallon inserts is used, not more than two holders loaded with 14 to 16 films should be placed into an insert simultaneously. A slight bending of the bottom of the film hanger toward the wall of the tank will help to prevent films from scraping against the wall.

The steps in the processing of the dental radiograph are: (1) development, (2) rinsing, (3) fixation, (4) washing, and (5) drying. Only two of these—development and fixation—generally involve chemicals.

The initial step in the processing sequence is the *development* of the film. This is done by slowly and completely immersing the film in the developer and gently agitating the hanger up and down a few times—taking care not to splash—to eliminate air bubbles from clinging to the film and allow the developer to make contact with all areas of the film. The handle of the film holder should rest on the lip of the insert. This permits the cover to be replaced. Set the activator arm on the timer and leave the film to develop until the timer goes off.

The next step in processing is *rinsing* the film. After the film is removed from the developer, one immerses the film hanger in the circulating water of the middle compartment for at least 30 seconds and agitates it so that the water can touch all the film. Even the tops of the handles of the hanger should be well rinsed to avoid transfer of developer into the fixer. Before being transferred to the fixer, the hanger should be held above the rinse water and allowed to drain for a few seconds to prevent carrying too much water into the fixer. The purpose of the rinsing is to remove as much of the alkaline developer as possible before placing the film in the fixer, thus preserving the acidity of the fixer and prolonging its useful life.

The next step after rinsing is the *fixation* of the film. One immerses the film and agitates it in the same manner as described for development. The timer is set and started—the common rule is to double the development time, and not less than 10 minutes. Unlike development time, fixing time is not too critical. Films may be left in the fixer for periods as long as an hour with perfect safety. Be sure to replace the cover to prevent oxidation.

When the radiograph is needed immediately for a quick reading of the x-ray image, the film may be read while it is still wet (wet reading). The film may be removed from the fixer as soon as it clears (usually after two or three minutes), should then be rinsed in water for a short interval and taken into the operatory for viewing; however, the film should be returned to the fixer as soon as possible to complete the fixation and permit further shrinking of the emulsion. If this is not done, some of the unexposed silver bromide grains may be left in the film, giving it a fogged and discolored appearance, and the emulsion may not harden completely.

The next step in processing is the *washing* of the film to remove chemicals left on the negative. This is done by placing the films in the circulating water of the rinse compartment for a minimum of 20 minutes. Longer washing is permissible but the film should always be removed not later than the end of the working day. If the temperature in the darkroom rises on a hot weekend or after the air conditioning is shut off, the water may become warm enough to melt the emulsion, leaving a film without an image. One should also be careful to ascertain that the rinse water is not much colder than the developer. This can cause *reticulation*, the formation of a network of cracks or wrinkles. The emulsion often cracks when subjected to variations in temperature from warm to cold.

The final step is the *drying* of the film. There are several ways to dry film: (1) Gently shake the water from the hanger and film, and suspend the hanger from a rod or drying rack, taking care that the film does not contact other films on adjacent racks or brush up against the walls; (2) follow the same procedure but use a fan or blower to expedite the drying, or (3) place the film in a heated drying cabinet, after shaking off the excess water. Films left in the cabinet too long, however, may become brittle. Always use a drip pan when moving the film hangers from the processing tank to the drying area and leave the pan under the film hanger until the film is dry.

The steps in the final procedures include: (1) checking to see that none of the films have loosened from the clip and dropped on the floor or the bottom of the tank; (2) cleaning up the work area to wipe up any moisture caused by dripping or accidental splashing of the water or solutions, and disposing of the film wrappings; (3) removing the dry films from the hangers and placing them in properly

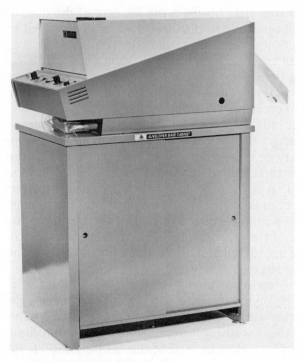

Fig. 8-7 An automatic processing unit equipped with temperature controls. This unit meters and circulates the required amounts of chemicals needed to process the films and makes it possible to process films in daylight. The film is inserted into the *Auveloper* through a slot in the top of the cabinet and is delivered completely processed through the chute in back 90 seconds later. (Courtesy of S. S. White Co., Dental Health Products Division.)

identified protective envelopes or on film mounts with identifying data. Film mounting techniques are discussed in the next chapter; and (4) removing or erasing identification markings from the hangers, and replacing hangers, the timer, or any equipment used in the proper place. At the end of the working day, drain the water compartment, turn off the water to the tank, and turn off all lights in the darkroom.

automatic processing

Recently a number of automatic film processing units have appeared on the market. These range from very small units designed to process only a single intraoral film at a time to very large and complex units that can process most types of intraoral and extraoral films (Fig. 8-7). Some of these units can produce a dry radiograph within 90 seconds. Automatic processing units are quite expensive and may on occasion require maintenance. As the cost decreases and the units become more trouble-free, they will probably find their way into more and more offices.

removal of processing stains from uniform

Despite all precautions, uniforms will occasionally become soiled with developer or fixer stains. Of the two, the developer is more difficult to remove. Never launder a uniform before trying to remove the spot. The best procedure is to rub a saturated soap solution into the spot as soon as possible, before it becomes permanently set into the fabric. Uniform shops and dental supply houses carry a number of very effective commercial spot removers. If such a remover is not available, the spot may be soaked for 5 or 10 minutes in a solution of a half ounce of household bleach and a half ounce of vinegar to a gallon of warm water, and then rinsed in plain water. Swabbing the area with fresh fixer may also be helpful. Stubborn stains may require longer soaking. After the spot is removed, the uniform should be laundered as soon as possible.

bibliography

Baker, Benjamin R., and Strickland, William D. *Dental Assisting, Course VII, Clinical Application,* 2d ed. Chapel Hill: University of North Carolina Press, 1971.

Ennis, Leroy M., Berry, Harrison M., and Phillips, James E. *Dental Roentgenology,* 6th ed. Philadelphia: Lea & Febiger, 1967.

Peterson, Shailer. *Clinical Dental Hygiene,* 3d ed. St. Louis: The C. V. Mosby Co., 1968.

Wilkins, Esther M. *Clinical Practice of the Dental Hygienist,* 3d ed. Philadelphia: Lea & Febiger, 1971.

Wuehrmann, Arthur M., and Manson-Hing, Lincoln R. *Dental Radiology,* 2d ed. St. Louis: The C. V. Mosby Co., 1969.

X-Rays in Dentistry, Rochester, N.Y.: Eastman Kodak Co., 1972.

9

identification

of anatomical landmarks

for mounting and interpretation

preliminary interpretation by auxiliary personnel

The complete interpretation of dental radiographs is the task of the dentist whose years of training and study have prepared him to render a diagnosis. However, according to the recent concept of expanded duties, a preliminary interpretation can be made by the trained dental auxiliary. The responsibility to finalize the diagnosis remains with the dentist.

The terms "interpretation" and "diagnosis" are often used interchangeably. This book, however, defines interpretation only as the ability to read the radiographs: diagnosis means the correlation of the patient's case history, clinical findings or test results, and radiographs. The dentist makes the diagnosis only after considering all the evidence pertaining to the patient's condition.

Because the dental auxiliary lacks the in-depth training of the dentist and can overlook important factors or err in interpretation, he must never express interpretative or diagnostic opinions to the patient. However, the dentist should encourage his assistant to make a private preliminary interpretation of the radiograph.

To produce consistently good radiographs, the student or auxiliary must not only be familiar with dental anatomy and exposure techniques but must know how to tell whether or not all desired information appears on the radiograph. He must know how to recognize anatomic landmarks and structures, as well as dental caries, restorative dentistry, periodontal disease, and uncomplicated periapical pathosis arising from tooth involvement.

This text can discuss only the common conditions. The study of complete interpretation of dental radiographs is far too complex to be feasible within the scope of this text for dental auxiliary personnel. Recognizing complex or uncommon pathological conditions is not the responsibility of the auxiliary. Several text books listed in the bibliography, particularly those by Bhaskar; Ennis, Berry, and Phillips; and Wuehrmann and Manson-Hing are excellent sources for reference and additional study. Although primarily written for the dental student and dentist, these books are liberally illustrated with helpful radiographs showing normal and abnormal structures and conditions of the jaws, the teeth, and the periodontium. With practice in identifying oral landmarks and structures, many learn to recognize all the common, and occasionally the less common, abnormalities. It is satisfying to have one's own analysis corroborated by the dentist's.

need to become familiar with anatomical landmarks

Before the auxiliary can arrange dental radiographs in meaningful sequence and secure each to its proper frame in the film mount, he must identify each separate tooth area portrayed. Most students enrolled in a radiography course will be simultaneously studying dental and cranial anatomy and have access to a skull and anatomy texts. The student should review the major landmarks of the face and the bony structures surrounding the teeth periodically until completely familiar with them and be able to identify them positively on a patient or radiograph.

In any text on anatomy, the illustrations show numerous protuberances, ridges, depressions, sutures, grooves, canals, and other landmarks. Only a portion of them are commonly used in dental radiography. Indeed, many are not visible on the average radiograph.

The prime concern of the auxiliary is to make use of a few of these to position film correctly, identify processed film, and make a correct preliminary interpretation.

significant anatomical landmarks

Only commonly used landmarks are labeled in illustrations in this chapter. Auxiliaries planning to work for certain specialists or in dental offices where highly sophisticated radiographic techniques are employed routinely will require additional training to recognize less common structures. Several of the texts mentioned in the preceding section are suited for advanced training.

Anatomical landmarks in this chapter are separated into the following groups: (1) landmarks of the face, (2) general landmarks of dental interest on the skull, (3) specific landmarks of the maxilla, and (4) specific landmarks of the mandible.

Facial Landmarks: The surface landmarks of the face cannot be distinguished on a radiograph; however, they help the radiographer to locate rapidly a number of important planes and structures. Such landmarks as the tip of the nose, the ala of the nose, the inner or outer canthus of the eye, the tragus of the ear, or the symphysis of the chin are often used in certain techniques for placing film and directing the PID. The positioning of the patient's head during intraoral radiography is often determined by aligning the mid-sagittal plane perpendicularly, and the ala-tragus plane parallel to the plane of the floor. Plane alignments and film positioning will be explained in Chapters 11 and 12.

Skull Landmarks: One can study the general landmarks of dental interest on the skull by comparing the labeling on the illustrations of the text used with their appearance on a dry skull. Most texts illustrate the anterior, lateral, and inferior aspects of the skull. You will find that the same landmark may be visible on more than one of these aspects. To make it easier to locate these landmarks, turn the skull so that it is oriented in the direction that corresponds to the illustration you are looking at.

Attempt to locate the following structures: the nasal bones, nasal spectum, the nasal fossa; the glenoid fossa and the acoustic meatus on the temporal bone; the mastoid process, the styloid process, the lateral pterygoid plate and the hamular process (hamulus) of the sphenoid bone; the zygomatic or malar bone, the zygomatic arch (zygoma), the maxilla, and the mandible.

Maxillary and Mandibular Landmarks: The dental radiographer is most concerned with the structures of the maxillae and the mandible because the teeth are located within the alveolar processes of these bones. It will help as you study these illustrations to remember that while the mandible is one bone, the maxillae are two bones, a right and left maxilla. Generally, but not always, the same structures appear on both sides.

Attempt to locate the following structures on the maxillae: the infraorbital foramen, the maxillary sinus (within the maxilla), the palatine process of the maxilla, the incisive (anterior palatine) foramen, the greater and lesser (posterior) palatine foramina, the median palatine suture. On the mandible, try to identify the body, the ramus, the inferior border, the angle of the mandible, the condyle, the coronoid process, the sigmoid (mandibular) notch, the mandibular canal, the mental foramen, the longual foreamen, the mental

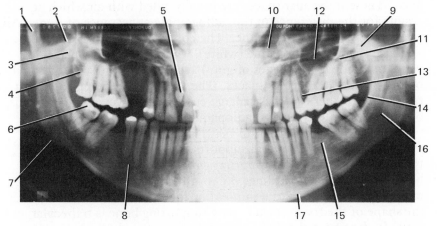

Fig. 9-1 Panoramic-type radiograph with landmarks indicated: 1. Condylar process; 2. sigmoid (mandibular) notch; 3. lateral pterygoid plate; 4. maxillary tuberosity; 5. supernumerary tooth; 6. metallic restorations; 7. angle of the mandible; 8. mental foramen; 9. coronoid process; 10. nasal cavity (fossa); 11. zygoma (malar bone); 12. maxillary sinus; 13. lamina dura; 14. external oblique ridge; 15. alveolar bone; 16. mandibular canal; 17. cortical bone forming inferior border of mandible. (Courtesy of UCLA School of Dentistry.)

ridge or process, the symphysis, the genial tubercles, the mylohyoid line or ridge, and the external oblique ridge.

The location of these structures of the skull, maxillae, and mandible should be memorized and identification should be practiced frequently. Some of the landmarks listed are visible only in the larger occlusal and extraoral radiographs. The number shown on any radiograph depends on the size of the film and the area exposed. Typical maxillary and mandibular structures, as well as some teeth and restorations, are identified in the 5 in. by 12 in. panoramic-type film shown (Fig. 9-1).

alveolar bone and tooth area

Before considering the specific structures visible in a full-mouth series of radiographs, a first step is to understand the normal bone and tooth structures. Although bones appear solid, they are solid only on the outside and are honeycombed within. Bone is classified as *compact bone*, a dense form of bone such as that which lines the outside layers of the maxillae and the mandible, and *trabecular* (cancellous) bone, which forms the bulk of the inner bone. Small, interconnected *trabeculae* (bars or plates of bone) form a multitude of various-sized compartments that account for the honeycomb appearance. These trabecular spaces are usually filled with air which accounts for the difference in the radiographic appearance of bone. All bone tissues appear radiopaque. The compact or cortical outer layers appear extremely radiopaque (white), whereas the trabecular bone varies in radiopacity (shades of gray) according to the size and number of the air-filled trabecular spaces. The area may even appear almost radiolucent if these spaces are large enough; however, in spite of this, bone is always described as radiopaque.

By definition, the *alveolar process* is that part of the maxilla or mandible that surrounds and supports the teeth. It is composed of the *lamina dura* and the *supporting bone*. The lamina dura is the hard, compact bone that lines the tooth socket (the alveolus). On radiographs, it appears as a thin radiopaque (white) line that outlines the shape of the tooth socket. The supporting bone is trabecular and varies in density in the different parts of the alveolar process.

The teeth are attached to the lamina dura by the fibers of the *periodontal* ligament (membrane) which is often so thin that it is not radiographically visible. When it can be seen, it has the appearance of a thin radiolucent (dark) border between the lamina dura and the roots of the teeth.

The tooth structures are enamel, dentin, cementum, and pulp. *Enamel*, the hardest body structure, covers the crown and is very radiopaque. The underlying *dentin* is not as dense, and appears less radiopaque. The *cementum* which covers the root is even less dense. Because only a thin layer of cementum covers the root, it is generally radiographically indistinguishable from the underlying dentin. Although all three highly calcified tooth structures vary in density and radiopacity, for descriptive purposes enamel, dentin, and cementum are considered radiopaque.

The *tooth pulp* that occupies the pulp chamber in the crown and the canals in the roots is the only noncalcified tooth tissue. As this soft tissue offers only minimal resistance to the passage of x-rays, it appears radiolucent. The end of the root canal is called the *apical foramen*. This foramen permits the entry and exit of nerves and blood vessels that nourish the tooth structures.

The development of carious lesions, periodontal disturbances, or pulpal disturbances or injuries can change the radiographic appearance of the structures described. Carious lesions (tooth decay) appear in the form of radiolucent areas in the coronal structures. Another degenerative process often seen on radiographs is horizontal and vertical bone loss. Horizontal bone loss is characterized by a relatively uniform reduction in the heights of the alveolar crest, whereas in vertical bone loss the height of the bone may be normal on one tooth and dip down almost to the apex of the next. Areas of bone loss appear radiolucent. Less frequently observed are abscesses and cysts (sac-like structures) that appear as radiolucent areas of various sizes and shapes in the areas surrounding the apical foramen.

In order to correctly identify and interpret the radiographs, one should also understand the dentition. A young child has 20 deciduous (baby or primary) teeth which are gradually lost as he gets older. During the transition years he has a mixed dentition—that is, both deciduous and permanent teeth. A radiograph may show several deciduous teeth, with partially resorbed roots, that are in the process of exfoliation as well as permanent teeth, whose roots are not yet fully formed, that are in the process of eruption. Such radiographs are often very difficult to identify and require the auxiliary to have a sound knowledge of dental anatomy. The permanent (secondary or succedaneous) teeth are 32 in number provided that all four of the third molars (wisdom teeth) are formed. Occasionally, teeth form but are unable to erupt; these are described as *impacted* teeth. Occasionally, a person may have extra teeth; such teeth are called *supernumerary* teeth. Another abnormality, the congenital absence of certain teeth, is described as *anodontia.*

Radiographs are normally exposed in four distinct areas of the maxillae: (1) the molar area (Fig. 9–2), (2) the premolar (bicuspid) area (Fig. 9–3), (3) the canine (cuspid) area (Fig. 9–4), and (4) the incisor area (Fig. 9–5). The normal structures visible in radiographs

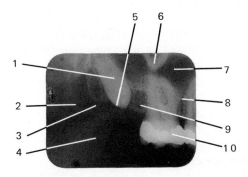

Fig. 9–2 Radiograph of a disto-angular view of the maxillary molar area. This radiograph has purposely been inserted further back in the molar area than is normally done in a routine examination. Some of the structures shown here only rarely appear on radiographs of this area: 1. Peg-shaped maxillary third molar; 2. hamular process (hamulus); 3. maxillary tuberosity; 4. coronoid process; 5. enamel of crown; 6. zygoma (malar bone); 7. maxillary sinus; 8. floor of maxillary sinus (white-radiopaque line); 9. cancellous alveolar bone; 10. metallic restoration.

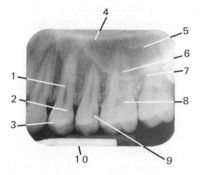

Fig. 9-3 Typical radiograph of maxillary premolar area: 1. Pulp canal; 2. dentin; 3. enamel of crown; 4. thin radiopaque line is septum dividing the maxillary sinus; 5. maxillary sinus; 6. lingual root of maxillary first molar; 7. anterior portion of zygoma or malar bone; 8. pulp chamber; 9. carious lesion; 10. large radiopaque area is outline of plastic biteblock.

of these areas vary in radiopacity or radiolucity in direct proportion to the densities of the exposed tissues. Each normal structure is identified at least once on the radiographs shown in Figures 9-2 through 9-5.

The following maxillary structures appear radiopaque: the *maxillary tuberosity,* a bone area behind the molars that is covered with the oral mucosa, marks the posterior limits of the maxillary arch; the *zygoma* (zygomatic arch), formed by processes of the zygomatic and temporal bones, is often seen in the premolar-molar area; the zygomatic (malar) bone is visible as a wide U-shaped band above the root areas of the first and second molars; the thin, dense bone forming the *floor* of the maxillary sinus is usually visible in the premolar-molar area; the thin *septum* (partition) that separates the nasal fossa from the maxillary sinus is often visible in the form of an inverted "Y" in the canine-premolar area; and the *nasal septum*, a thin dense bone structure that separates the right nasal fossa from the left, may be visible in the incisor area. Although not a maxillary structure, the tip of the *coronoid process* of the mandible, to which the temporalis muscle attaches, and the hamulus (hamular process) of the sphenoid

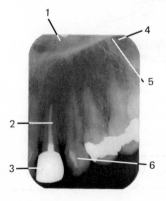

Fig. 9-4 Typical radiograph of the maxillary canine area: 1. Nasal fossa; 2. root canal filling (probably gutta percha); 3. metal crown (probably gold with a porcelain front); 4. maxillary sinus; 5. typical inverted "Y" formation of the maxillary sinus formed at junction of the floor of the nasal fossa and the anterior wall of the maxillary sinus; 6. radiopaque area is remnant of zinc phosphate type cement base (remainder of restoration has broken off or disintegrated).

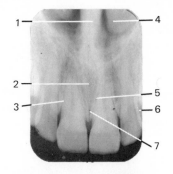

Fig. 9-5 Typical radiograph of the maxillary incisor area: 1. Nasal septum; 2. incisive foramen; 3. radiolucent line next to root is space occupied by periodontal membrane; 4. nasal fossa; 5. radiopaque line outlining the alveolus is the lamina dura; 6. radiopaque area is caused by overlap of canine over lateral incisor; 7. median palatine suture.

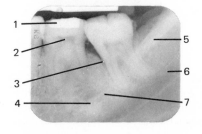

Fig. 9-6 Typical mandibular molar area: 1. Metal restoration; 2. pulp chamber; 3. vertical bone resorption (periodontia); 4. condensing osteitis—radiopaque area; 5. external oblique line—diagonal radiopaque band; 6. mandibular canal—a wide radiolucent diagonal area; 7. mylohyoid ridge—diagonal radiopaque band about 2–3 mm below external oblique line.

bone, a hook-like structure that serves as a muscle tendon attachment, are occasionally visible in the maxillary molar area.

The following maxillary structures are radiolucent: the *maxillary sinus*, a large air chamber in the maxilla, visible in the areas from the canine to the molars; the *nasal fossa*, a large air space divided by the nasal septum, is often visible above the incisors; the *incisive foramen* (anterior palatine), a round or pear shaped opening that varies greatly in size, serves for the passage of nerves and blood vessels and is often visible near or between the apices of the central incisors (this foramen is occasionally mistaken for an abscess formation); and the *median palatine suture*, a thin line that delineates the midline of the palate and the junction of the right and left maxilla, is frequently seen in the incisor area.

The mandibular areas normally exposed are the same as those of the maxillae: (1) the molar area (Fig. 9–6), (2) the premolar area (Fig. 9–7), (3) the canine area (Fig. 9–8), and (4) the incisor area (Fig. 9–9). Each normal structure on the radiographs in Figures 9–6 through 9–9 is identified at least once.

The following mandibular structures appear radiopaque: the *external oblique line* (ridge), a heavy crest of bone serving for muscle attachments extends at an angle from the ramus down the lateral surface of the body to a point near the mental foramen and can be seen in the premolar-molar areas; the *mylohyoid line* (ridge), another diagonal crest of bone for muscle attachments on the lingual side that

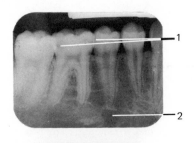

Fig. 9-7 Typical radiograph of mandibular premolar area: 1. Incipient caries (radiolucent); 2. mental foramen.

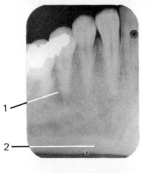

Fig. 9-8 Typical radiograph of mandibular canine area: 1. Mental foramen; 2. dense cortical bone forming inferior border of mandible (radiopaque).

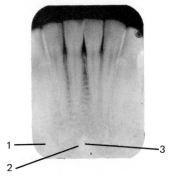

Fig. 9-9 Typical radiograph of mandibular incisor area: 1. Mental ridge or process (a diagonal slightly radiopaque area); 2. genial tubercles appear as small circular radiopaque area; 3. lingual foramen appears as tiny radiolucent area in center of the genial tubercles.

parallels the external oblique line, can often be seen just slightly below and parallel to the external oblique line in the premolar-molar areas; the *mental ridge* (protuberance), a triangular prominence on the lateral surface of the body, is visible in the canine area; the *inferior border of the mandible,* a heavy layer or cortical bone, may be visible if the radiograph was deeply depressed into the mouth; and the *genial tubercles*, four small bony crests on the lingual surface that serve for muscle attachments, may be visible at the midline below the apices of the central incisors.

The following mandibular areas appear radiolucent: the *mandibular canal*, a canal for the passage of the mandibular nerve and blood vessels, is outlined by very thin layers of cortical bone and can be seen in the premolar-molar areas below the apices of the teeth; the *mental foramen*, a small circular opening on the lateral side of the body, is often seen near the apices of the premolars; and the *lingual foramen*, a very small circular area surrounded by the genial tubercles, may occasionally be seen in the central incisor area but is often so small that it goes unnoticed.

It should be kept in mind that dental radiographs are two-dimensional shadow pictures of three-dimensional objects. Depending on the relationship of the angle of the central ray to the structure, and the angle at which the film is positioned in relationship to the structures, two or more radiographs of the same area may show the identical structures to be of different size or in a slightly different position. Occasionally, a structure clearly visible on one film cannot be located on another film of the same area for this reason. Moreover, some anatomic structures or landmarks may be absent on some persons or present on only one side (a technique which is based on exposing radiographs of the same area at different angles is sometimes used to locate the position of imbedded objects). There is also a variation in the radiolucency of the soft tissues. The outline of the mucosa that covers the alveolar bone can usually be discerned as a thin outline above the crest of the alveolar bone. The lips and cheeks can seldom be distinguished; however, a shadow of the lip outline or the tip of the nose is sometimes visible. Given a correctly exposed and processed radiograph, the auxiliary should have little trouble recognizing landmarks and structures—especially after a bit of practice.

mounting the radiographs

Mounting is extremely important so that each of a series of radiographs can be arranged in proper anatomic relationship to all other radiographs exposed on a patient at a given time. Correct mounting helps to eliminate embarrassing errors caused by confusing radiographs of the patient's right with the left side. When mounted, radiographs are easier to view and interpret.

Film mounts are celluloid, cardboard, or plastic holders with frames or windows for the radiographs. Attaching the radiographs to the film mounts is called mounting. Film mounts are available in many sizes and with numerous combinations of windows or frames to fit films of different sizes. Most mounts are large enough to accommodate a full-mouth series of radiographs although some hold only a few or even a single radiograph. Standard ready-made mounts are used in most dental offices; however, several firms will make custom mounts to suit special needs.

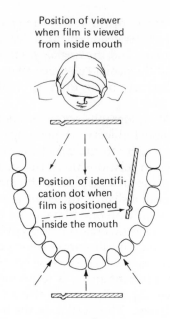

Position of viewer
when film is viewed
from inside mouth

Position of identifi-
cation dot when
film is positioned
inside the mouth

Position of viewer when
film is viewed from
recommended position
outside of mouth

Fig. 9–10 Regardless of the tooth area involved, whenever an x-ray film is positioned in the mouth, the raised portion of the identification dot (the convexity) must face the x-ray tube and the source of radiation. Therefore, when the film is viewed from outside the mouth or from in front of the patient, the convex part of the dot faces the viewer.

The task of mounting the radiographs is not difficult once the novice becomes familiar with the appearance of the anatomic structures and masters a few simple procedures. First, he must be able to distinguish which films are of the patient's right and which of the left side. A little identification dot near the edge of the film appears convex or concave depending upon the side from which the film is viewed. When the film is mounted with the convex dot toward you, the patient's left side is on your right (Fig. 9–10).

Two systems of film mounting are commonly used. Some dentists prefer to have the radiographs mounted so that they give the effect of viewing the patient from behind. In this arrangement the concave dot faces the viewer. Other dentists prefer the opposite method, in which the film is viewed from a point outside the patient. The convex part of the dot is then toward the viewer. In an effort to achieve standardization, the ADA recommends the latter method.

Mounting generally refers only to intraoral films. The large extraoral films are already identified through the use of metal lettering and are usually placed in a protective envelope. The patient's name and the date of the exposure are always written on the outside of these envelopes. Occasionally, single intraoral radiographs are not mounted but are slipped into a coin envelope and attached to the record card. However, it is better to mount even single or small groups of radiographs; a full-mouth series should always be mounted for easier and faster viewing. Obviously, each film mount must be identified with at least the patient's name, case number if applicable, and the date. Few things are as useless in a dental office as unidentifiable radiographs.

The auxiliary generally follows a routine when mounting a set of radiographs. First, he washes his hands to prevent smudging the films and lays a clean towel over the workbench in front of an illuminator. To avoid confusing radiographs, he removes only one patient's films from the clips of the film hanger at one time (sometimes films of different patients are processed on the same hanger). He then arranges the films so that all the identification dots face in the same direction—either toward the viewer or toward the towel. The former is preferred, but either method is acceptable as long as all the dots face the same way.

The radiographs must be arranged just as the teeth in the mouth are; the anterior teeth must be mounted in the middle frames and the posterior teeth in the frames on either side of the mount. The maxillary teeth must be positioned so that the incisal edges or occlusal surfaces point downward and the root upward. The mandibular teeth are mounted the opposite way, with the incisal or occlusal surfaces pointing up and the roots pointing to the bottom of the mount.

Several distinctive tooth characteristics and bone structures make mounting easier: (1) the roots and crowns of the maxillary anterior teeth are larger than those of the mandibular teeth; (2) the maxillary molars generally have three roots, the mandibular molars only two; (3) most roots curve toward the distal; (4) the large radiolucent areas denoting the nasal fossa or the maxillary sinus indicate that the radiograph is of a maxillary area; (5) the radiolucent mental foramen indicates that the film belongs in the mandibular canine-premolar area; and (6) the body of the mandible has a distinct upward curve toward the ramus in the molar area.

With these characteristics firmly in mind, the auxiliary holds the radiographs up to the illuminator and separates them into three groups: (1) the anterior films, (2) the posterior films, and (3) interproximal films. The radiographs of each of these groups is then identified as right or left, maxillary or mandibular. They are put into the proper order and placed on the mount one by one. The auxiliary should handle films by their edges to avoid smudging them. After mounting the last radiograph, he checks the entire film mount carefully to make sure that no films were reversed accidentally or mounted upside down, and that the name and date are on the mount.

The method just described is particularly recommended for beginners. As their skills increase, many auxiliaries develop simpler and faster techniques.

film viewing

The importance of using a good illuminated view box for mounting and interpreting the radiographs cannot be overemphasized. Many types of view box are available, both built-ins and portables. The preferred type for dental office use has a dark nonreflective frame, a frosted glass panel, and a rheostat to vary the intensity of the light (Fig. 9–11). Blocking out excess light reduces glare and facilitates viewing. The use of black cardboard or frosted film mounts also helps to reduce glare and enhances the detail of the images.

Some viewers are also equipped with a magnifying device. A new product (which unfortunately is rather expensive) is an enhancer. This combines the principles of a camera equipped with a zoom lens with those of a television screen. By changing range, focus, or light intensity, this device permits the viewer to examine the magnified radiograph in minute detail.

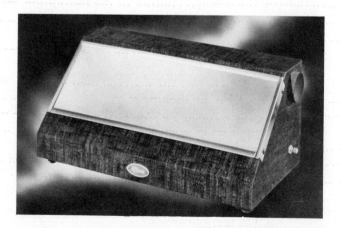

Fig. 9–11 This desk viewer has two levels of light to permit better diagnosis. A view box with variable light control makes it possible to diminish glare and to secure the maximum information from the radiographs because the tooth and bone structures may be enhanced when the light is varied. In some dental installations, the view boxes are built into the walls of the operatories and/or darkrooms. (Courtesy of Rinn Corporation, Dental X-Ray Division.)

Mounted radiographs show the relations between major tooth areas and reveals each in its entirety, clearly and with a minimum of distortion. If circumstances permit, substandard radiographs should be retaken before being submitted to the dentist. Depending on the auxiliary's status and responsibility in the dental office, he may now proceed to make a preliminary interpretation and discuss it with the dentist. After this, the film mount should be placed in a properly identified protective envelope and filed until needed at the patient's next visit.

radiographic interpretation of the teeth and periodontium

Besides recognizing structures and landmarks, the auxiliary must be able to identify the normal tooth tissues, the various commonly used restorative materials, common lesions and pathological conditions, fractures, impactions, or tooth abnormalities, early stages of tooth development and eruption, and calculus.

The radiographic appearance of normal tooth structures was discussed earlier in the chapter. These are identified easily by most auxiliaries. The differentiation between the various restorative materials is a little more difficult and requires additional experience.

Some restorative materials are easy to identify; others can be differentiated only by the size and contour of the restoration, its probable location on the tooth, and the relative degree of radiopacity or radiolucency.

For example, the image outlines of all metal restorations of approximately equal density appear extremely radiopaque. Thus it is impossible to determine whether the material used was gold, silver, or a base metal alloy. Only by looking at the size and contour of the restoration is it possible to make an educated guess based on what materials are generally used in such circumstances. Further, it is not always possible to determine on which tooth surface the restoration is located. A filling looks the same whether it is on the facial or lingual side of the tooth because radiographs are merely shadow pictures. The image of a restoration on one surface may be superimposed on the image of a larger restoration giving the appearance of only one restoration instead of two or even more. Some materials, such as cements used in dentistry, can be differentiated only by the location on the tooth and the degree of radiopacity, while esthetic restorations, such as fused porcelain, silicate, and the acrylic resins (plastic) appear quite similar and exhibit only slight differences in radiolucency. Of these three, fused porcelain is the densest and least radiolucent, while the acrylic resins are least dense and most radiolucent. Thus, it should be obvious that a visual and digital examination is required to verify the conditions shown on a radiograph.

All metals used in dentistry, whether in the form of fillings, crowns, bridges, or orthodontic wires, the gutta percha points used in root canals, the zinc phosphate cements used in bases and for cementation, the zinc oxide-eugenol pastes used as protective bases, and those composite filling materials and calcium hydroxide pastes used in pulp capping that have opaque materials added to them exhibit some degree of radiopacity and are described as radiopaque.

The fused porcelains used for crowns and as facings for bridgework, the silicates used for filling anterior teeth, the acrylic resins used for fillings and crowns, most composite fillings, and most calcium hydroxide pastes exhibit some degree of radiolucency and are described as radiolucent. Several of these materials, as well as some common lesions and structures, are identified on the radiographs in Figures 9–12 through 9–16.

Most common lesions and pathologic conditions of the teeth are radiolucent; however, those that involve structural growth or calcification are radiopaque. Examples of such conditions are: *hypercementosis*, a pathologic overgrowth of the cementum; *condensing osteitis*, a thickening of the trabecular spaces in some areas of the bones;

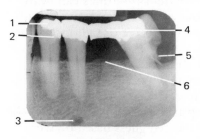

Fig. 9–12 Mandibular premolar-molar area: 1. Metal restoration—probably amalgam or gold (radiopaque); 2. zinc phosphate cement base under restoration (slightly less radiopaque); 3. mental foramen (radiolucent); 4. bridge—gold (radiopaque); 5. resorption of distal root of molar (radiolucent); 6. horizontal bone loss caused by periodontal condition (bone recession of about 6 mm).

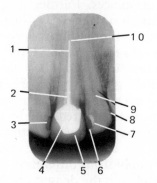

Fig. 9–13 Maxillary incisor area: 1. Gutta percha root canal filling (radiopaque); 2. pulp canal paste of zinc oxide-eugenol type (less radiopaque); 3. silicate restoration (radiolucent); 4. gold core under porcelain jacket crown (radiopaque); 5. porcelain fused to gold core (relatively radiolucent); 6. acrylic restoration (radiolucent); 7. zinc phosphate cement base under acrylic restoration (radiopaque); 8. incipient caries (radiolucent); 9. pulp canal; 10. root apex—root canal not completely filled to apex.

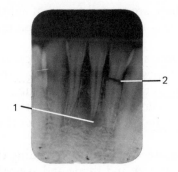

Fig. 9-14 Mandibular incisor area: 1. Radicular cyst (radiolucent); 2. fractured lateral incisor (fracture line is radiolucent).

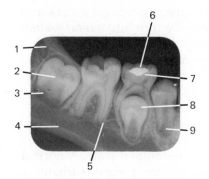

Fig. 9-15 Mixed dentition in the mandibular molar-premolar area: 1. Enamel organ of second permanent molar seen as radiopaque outline within radiolucent tooth follicle; 2. unerupted permanent second molar; 3. remnant of tooth follicle (thin radiolucent area around second molar crown); 4. inferior border of mandible (radiopaque); 5. almost complete apex of permanent first molar—radiolucent area will remain until root formation is complete; 6. amalgam restoration (radiopaque); 7. deciduous second molar; 8. crown of permanent second premolar starting to resorb roots of the deciduous second molar; 9. incomplete root formation of erupting permanent first premolar.

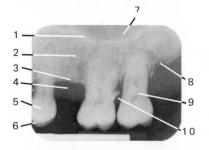

Fig. 9-16 Maxillary molar area: 1. Thin radiolucent line marks inferior border of the maxillary sinus; 2. extraction site—bone being regenerated; 3. alveolar crest—severe horizontal bone loss; 4. gingiva—soft tissue (slightly radiolucent); 5. dentin (radiopaque); 6. enamel (heavier radiopaque than the dentin); 7. maxillary sinus (radiolucent); 8. site of third molar extration—bone not filled in completely; 9. pulp stone within pulp chamber (radiopaque); 10. calculus formation (radiopaque) accompanied by periodontal involvement and bone loss.

exostosis (torus), a bony growth projecting outward from a bone or over a tooth area; *osteomas*, hard tumors developing on bone; and *odontomas*, tumors of toothlike structures. *Dental calculus*, although not classified as a lesion because its formation is a normal process for many persons, is a gradual deposition of calcium and other inorganic salts and organic matter around the gingival areas of the teeth. The accumulation and growth of these calculus deposits contributes to periodontal disturbances. Although there are several forms of supra-gingival and subgingival calculus, all forms appear radiopaque on the radiographs.

Dental caries are the radiolucent lesions most frequently encountered on radiographs. These are three types: (1) *incipient caries,* the small breaks in the enamel often visible in the areas between the teeth; (2) *recurrent caries,* decay that occurs under the restoration or around the margins; and (3) *rampant decay,* the deep cavities that are easiest to recognize.

Less common than caries are the radiolucent areas surrounding the apices of the teeth. These vary greatly in size and shape and are called abscesses, granulomas, or cysts. They are difficult to differentiate by radiographs alone. As a rule, *acute abscesses* (early stages of pulpal or periapical infection) are barely discernible, becoming more radiolucent as they become chronic. These appear as a circular dark area around the apex. Chronic abscesses usually turn into *dental granulomas*, masses of granulation tissue usually surrounded by a fibrous sac continuous with the periodontal membrane and attached to the root apex. Many types of *dental cysts* are known. *Radicular cysts* may have a well-defined outline of cortical bone. *Residual cysts* often appear as radiolucencies at extraction sites.

The destruction of the lamina dura, with the resultant widening of the periodontal membrane and radiolucent areas indicating horizontal and vertical bone loss, typifies periodontal disease. A normal condition that the beginner often mistakes for a bone disturbance is the *eruption cyst,* a radiolucent sac (follicle) frequently observed surrounding the tooth germ or erupting tooth. This radiolucent area disappears after the tooth erupts.

Other radiolucencies frequently encountered include: *fracture lines,* thin lines that delineate a bone or tooth fracture; *rarefying osteitis,* a bone disease in which the inorganic matter is lessened; and *resorption,* which may take two forms—(1) normal resorption such as happens when the roots of the deciduous teeth are resorbed, and (2) pathologic resorption, a process in which disease or unusual pressures cause the resorption of bone or the roots of the permanent teeth.

Solid structures embedded within the dental arches, such as un-erupted teeth, impacted teeth, supernumerary teeth, broken root fragments, or foreign particles, appear radiopaque and are generally identifiable by shape or contour. These should not pose any serious problem in identification.

The foregoing is only a partial list of structures or lesions that may be visible on radiographs, and any attempt to describe them fully belongs in a text on radiographic interpretation. The dental auxiliary who attempts to make a preliminary interpretation must bear in mind that many of the lesions described look similar. Only the dentist can differentiate between these after evaluating the clinical signs and symptoms. Even then, he may need a biopsy report to determine the exact type of lesion encountered on the radiograph.

filing and storage of dental radiographs

After the radiographs are mounted they should be placed in a protective envelope and given to the dentist so that he can examine them before discussing them with the patient. The radiographs should be in the operating room along with other records each time the patient visits the office.

After the appointment, the radiographs should be filed away and stored until needed again. They may be stored along with the record folder or in a separate x-ray filing cabinet. The radiographs may be filed by either name or case number, as long as they can be located rapidly when needed. The need for an orderly filing system cannot be overstressed; missing radiographs can be a source of much annoyance. Some dentists store current radiographs in one file and older ones in another. When new radiographs are exposed, the old ones are often removed from the mounts and placed into smaller identified and dated envelopes to conserve space.

All radiographs should be handled with care to prevent smudging or scratching and should be protected from heat damage by storage in cool, well-ventilated areas. Although radiographs are seldom used after more than six months or a year because oral conditions change constantly in most patients, they are valuable for comparing present with previous conditions. Sometimes they are needed in a court of law. Therefore the dentist should preserve them until he is certain that the statute of limitations for his state has expired.

bibliography

Bhasker, S. N. *Roentgenographic Interpretation for the Dentist,* St. Louis: The C. V. Mosby Co., 1970.

Ennis, Leroy M., Berry, Harrison M., and Phillips, James E. *Dental Roentgenology,* 6th ed. Philadelphia: Lea & Febiger, 1967.

O'Brien, Richard C. *Dental Radiography,* 2d ed. Philadelphia: W. B. Saunders Co., 1972.

Peterson, Shailer. *Clinical Dental Hygiene,* 3d ed. St. Louis: The C. V. Mosby Co., 1968.

Schwarzrock, Shirley Pratt, and Jensen, James R. *Effective Dental Assisting*, 4th ed. Dubuque, Iowa: William C. Brown Co., 1973.

Wilkins, Esther M. *Clinical Practice of the Dental Hygienist*, 3d ed. Philadelphia: Lea & Febiger, 1971.

Wuehrmann, Arthur M., and Manson-Hing, Lincoln R. *Dental Radiology*, 2d ed. St. Louis: The C. V. Mosby Co., 1969.

10
identifying and correcting
faulty radiographs

importance of identifying faulty radiographs

It is important to be able to tell when a radiograph is inadequate and to understand why. Only clear, properly processed radiographs with minimal distortion of the image have diagnostic value to the dentist. Any radiograph that does not meet that standard should be retaken if possible. Being aware of the causes of inadequacies and the methods of correcting them should prevent repetition of mistakes.

inadequacies caused by faulty exposure techniques

Most faulty radiographs are caused by errors in exposure technique, such as incorrect positioning of the film packet, incorrect positioning of the tube head and PID, or incorrect exposure factors. Of course, position errors may also mean that the patient moved his head after the film, tube head and PID were in place or allowed the film to slip. The radiographer must always caution the patient not to move his head and to hold the film firmly. A small booklet, *Radiodontic Pitfalls*, is available from the Eastman Kodak Company.

Inadequacies Attributable to Incorrect Positioning of the Film

1. *Absence of Apical Structures* (Figs. 10–1 and 10–6)
Probable cause: Film not placed high enough in patient's mouth.
Correction: Raise the film in patient's mouth.

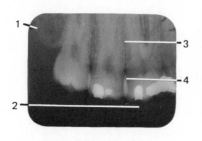

Fig. 10-1 Radiograph of maxillary molar: 1. Radiograph is too dark. It was overexposed and also possibly overdeveloped; 2. excessive occlusal margin with resultant absence of the complete apical structures caused by film being placed too low in mouth; 3. tooth structures are elongated because the vertical angulation was insufficiently steep; 4. overlapping in the proximal areas because in horizontal angulation the central beam was not directed through the interproximal spaces at right angles to the mean tangent of the buccal surfaces.

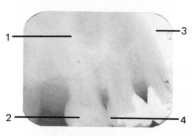

Fig. 10-2 Radiograph of maxillary molar area: 1. Light image caused by underexposure or underdevelopment; 2. absence of occlusal margin or all coronal structures—film was placed too high in mouth; 3. cone cut—an unexposed area caused by faulty centering of the PID; 4. overlap in interproximal area traceable to faulty horizontal angulation.

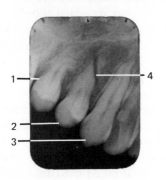

Fig. 10-3 Radiograph of maxillary canine area: 1. Extreme foreshortening of the image caused by excessive (too steep) vertical angulation; 2. slanting or diagonal occlusal plane caused by poor positioning of film; 3. canine not in center of film. This tooth, instead of the first premolar, should be the center of diagnostic interest in this particular area; 4. black pressure mark due to excessive pressure or bend in the film which broke the film emulsion.

2. *Absence of Coronal Structures* (Fig. 10-2)
Probable cause: Film not placed low enough in patient's mouth.
Correction: Lower the film in patient's mouth.

3. *Absence of Mesial Structures*
Probable cause: Film was placed too far back in patient's mouth.
Correction: Move the film mesially (toward midline).

4. *Absence of Distal Structures*
Probable cause: Film was placed too far forward in patient's mouth.
Correction: Move the film distally (toward back of mouth).

5. *Slanting or Diagonal Instead of Straight Occlusal Plane* (Fig. 10-3)
Probable cause: Edge of film was not parallel with incisal or occlusal plane of the teeth.

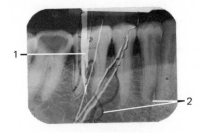

Fig. 10-4 Radiograph of mandibular molar-premolar area: 1. White streaks caused by scratching the soft emulsion with the clips of other film holders in the processing tanks; 2. dark line indicates where film was bent.

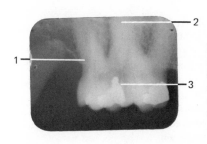

Fig. 10-5 Radiograph of maxillary incisor area: 1. Film was accidentally reversed when placed in mouth resulting in a very light image and the appearance of a characteristic herringbone or diamond pattern; 2. the central beam was not directed toward the center of the film resulting in an area which was not exposed and appears as a semicircular cone cut.

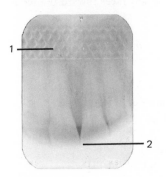

Fig. 10-6 Radiograph of maxillary molar area: 1. Poor definition. Image is blurred and distorted by excessive movement of tube head or patient during exposure; 2. lack of complete apical structures. Film was placed too low and also too far distally; 3. overlapping of structures caused by faulty horizontal angulation.

Correction: Straighten the film packet. The use of a cotton roll between the film and the tooth may make this easier.

6. *Vertical Instead of Horizontal Film Placement in Posterior Areas*
Probable cause: Film was placed with its longest dimension vertically. This is seldom desirable in posterior areas.
Correction: Rotate the film so that the widest dimension is placed horizontally and film edge is parallel with occlusal plane.

7. *Horizontal Instead of Vertical Film Placement in Anterior Areas*
Probable cause: Film was placed with its widest dimension horizontally. Such placement is undesirable and produces major dimensional distortion of the image.
Correction: Rotate the film so that the longest dimension is placed vertically. The short edge of the film should be placed parallel to the incisal edges of the anterior teeth.

8.   *Bent Film Packet* (Fig. 10–4)
Probable cause: Curvature of palate or lingual arch and strong finger pressure on film.
Correction: Place cotton roll behind teeth in area of greatest curvature and ask patient to reduce finger pressure. Consider the use of a film holder and narrower film.

9.   *Diamond or Herringbone Pattern* (Fig. 10–5)
Probable cause: Film was reversed and back side was facing teeth and the radiation source.
Correction: Turn the film so that the tube side faces toward the teeth and the radiation source.

Inadequacies Attributable to Incorrect Positioning of the Tube Head or PID

1.   *Elongation of Image* (Fig. 10–1)
Probable cause: Insufficient vertical angulation of the PID.
Correction: Increase the vertical angulation. Also check position of film and patient's head.

2.   *Foreshortening of the Image* (Fig. 10–3)
Probable cause: Excessive vertical angulation of the PID.
Correction: Decrease the vertical angulation. Also check position of film and patient's head.

3.   *Overlapping of the Image* (Figs. 10–1, 10–2, and 10–6)
Probable cause: Incorrect rotation of tube head and PID in horizontal plane. Superimposition of the images of proximal surfaces occurs when the central beam is not directed perpendicularly toward the film through the interproximal spaces.
Correction: Depending on the direction of the overlapping, maintain the vertical angulation but change the horizontal angulation of the PID either toward the mesial or distal as required to enable the central beam to pass through the interproximal embrasures.

4.   *Cone Cut* (Figs. 10–2 and 10–5)
Probable cause: The primary beam of radiation was not directed toward the center of the film and did not completely expose all parts of the film.
Correction: Maintain horizontal and vertical angulation and move the tube head either up, down, mesially, or distally depending upon which area of the radiograph shows a clear unexposed area.

Inadequacies Attributable to Exposure Factors

1.   *Light (thin) Image* (Fig. 10–2)
Probable cause: Insufficient exposure time in relation to milliamperage, kilovoltage, and distance selected. May also be caused by insufficient time in developer, weak or oxidized developer, or reversed film.

Correction: Increase the exposure time, the milliamperage, the kilovoltage, or a combination of these factors.

2. *Dark Image* (Fig. 10–1)

Probable cause: Overexposure (excessive mAs, kVp, or too short target-film distance). Alternate cause—too long in developer.

Correction: Decrease the exposure time, the milliamperage, the kilovoltage, or a combination of these factors.

3. *Absence of Image*

Probable cause: Failure to turn on line switch or to maintain firm pressure on activator button during the exposure. Alternate causes—electrical failure or malfunction of the x-ray machine or processing errors (placing film in fixer first or having the emulsion dissolve in warm rinse water).

Correction: Turn on x-ray machine and maintain firm pressure on activator button during entire exposure period.

Inadequacies Attributable to Miscellaneous Errors in Exposure Technique

1. *Poor Definition* (Fig. 10–6)

Probable cause: Movement during exposure. Caused by patient movement, film slippage, or vibration of tube head and PID.

Correction: Steady tube head before starting exposure. Ask patient to maintain steady pressure on film and not to move.

2. *Double Image*

Probable cause: Accidentally exposing the same film twice.

Correction: Place exposed film into film safe immediately.

3. *Superimposed Image*

Probable cause: Failure to first examine the mouth and remove any appliances such as removable bridges, partial or full dentures, and space maintainers.

Correction: Look in patient's mouth and remove any appliance.

4. *Pressure Marks (black streaks)* (Fig. 10–3)

Probable cause: Bending or excessive pressure that causes film emulsion to crack.

Correction: Avoid excess pressure on film. Do not bend film except for minimal softening of corners to avoid hurting the patient with the sharp edges of the film packet.

5. *Wrapping Paper Stuck to Film*

Probable cause: Break in wrapping by rough handling enabled saliva to penetrate to the emulsion. Moisture softened the emulsion causing the black paper to stick to the film.

Correction: Careful handling prevents break in the seal of the film packet. Always blot moisture from film packet after removing it from the mouth.

inadequacies caused by faulty processing techniques

Another major cause of faulty radiographs can be traced to errors in the processing technique. Many of these, such as misreading the temperature on the thermometer, forgetting to wind or set the timer, setting the timer incorrectly, failure to remove the film from the developer when the timer rings, and damage to the emulsion by handling or by chemical contamination, can be blamed on haste or carelessness.

Inadequacies Attributable to Failure to Follow the Suggested Time-Temperature Cycle

1. *Light Image* (Fig. 10–2)
Probable cause: Underdevelopment—film not left in developer long enough. The colder the developer, the longer the time required. Alternate causes—weakened developer or underexposure.
Correction: Check temperature of developer and consult time-temperature chart before placing film in developer. If necessary, fill the inserts with fresh solutions.

2. *Dark Image*
Probable cause: Overdevelopment—film left in developer too long. The warmer the developer, the less time is required. Alternate cause—overexposure to radiation.
Correction: Check temperature of developer and consult time-temperature chart before placing film in developer.

3. *Absence of Image*
Probable cause: Film was placed in fixer before being placed in developer or emulsion may have dissolved in warm rinse water. Alternate cause—film may not have been exposed.
Correction: Place film in developer first and promptly remove film at end of washing period.

Inadequacies Caused by Faulty Handling of the Film

1. *Smudged Film*
Probable cause: Fingermarks on the dry film or on the soft wet emulsion.
Correction: Avoid contact with surface of radiograph. Handle films carefully and by the edges only. Hands should be clean and free of moisture.

2. *Torn Film*
Probable cause: Too much haste in unwrapping film packet.
Correction: Unwrap film packet carefully.

3. *Thin Black Lines*
Probable cause: Static electricity was produced when film was pulled out of wrapping too fast.
Correction: Pull film out of wrapping slowly.

4. *White Lines or Marks* (Fig. 10-4)
Probable cause: Film was scratched while the emulsion was soft by a
sharp object such as a film clip or film hanger. Scratching removes the
emulsion from the base.
Correction: Be careful when inserting a second film hanger into an
insert. Avoid contact with other films or hangers.

5. *Black Image*
Probable cause: Film accidentally exposed to white light or exposed
for a long period in warm developer.
Correction: Turn off all light in darkroom except proper safelight before unwrapping film. Lock door or warn others to stay out by turning
on the "in-use" sign.

6. *Partial Image*
Probable cause: The level of the developer was too low to cover the
entire film.
Correction: Replenish the processing solutions to the proper level or
fasten the films to lower clips on the hanger.

7. *Clear Areas on Film*
Probable cause: Films stuck together in developer, so developer was
not able to act on both sides of the film emulsion. Alternate cause—
attaching two films to a clip through failure to separate films in two-
film packets.
Correction: Agitate films gently when inserting into the developer—
make certain that films do not touch those on other hangers.

8. *Dark or Opaque Areas on Film* (Fig. 10-7)
Probable cause: Films stuck together in fixer. The fixer was not able
to neutralize the developer in those areas and development continues
partially.
Correction: Agitate films gently when inserting into the developer—
make certain the films do not come in contact with those on other
hangers.

9. *Reticulation*
Probable cause: Temperature of processing solutions too hot, or there
is too great a difference between the temperature of the processing
solutions and the rinse water. Temperature differences of ten degrees

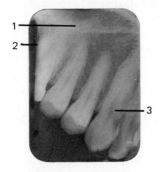

Fig. 10-7 Radiograph of maxillary canine
area: 1. Rusty or brown stain covering entire
radiograph caused by improper washing after
fixing; 2. thin dark area along side of film
caused by two films touching in fixer with
failure to stop the action of the developer;
3. positioning error. Canine not in center of
film with resultant loss of apical structure and
a diagonal occlusal plane.

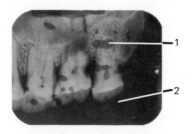

Fig. 10–8 Radiograph of maxillary molar area: 1. Dark spots on radiograph caused by premature contact of film surface with developer splashed on workbench. Bench should always be clean; 2. uneven occlusal margin caused by poor film positioning.

Fig. 10–9 Radiograph of mandibular premolar-molar area: 1. Entire radiograph is fogged with a resultant lack of contrast. Fog may be caused by overage film (as in radiograph shown), storage, exposure to radiation or light, contaminated chemicals, or numerous other causes; 2. radiograph was also poorly centered and positioned. The film was depressed too far in the mouth and does not show all of the occlusal cusps and the film was positioned too far back to be satisfactory as a premolar film and too far forward enough to show the distal roots of the molar.

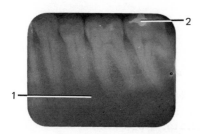

may cause the film to become pitted and reticulated through the softening and melting of the emulsion.

Correction: Determine that the temperature in the processing solutions is approximately the same as that of the rinse water. Do not begin to process the film until the circulating water has cooled or warmed the developer and fixer. Temperatures in excess of 80 degrees should be avoided.

10. *Curled Films*
Probable cause: Too rapid drying of film through use of heat.
Correction: Slower, more gradual drying. Avoid prolonged drying in electric dryer.

11. *Scratched Film*
Probable cause: Failure to protect dried radiograph.
Correction: Careful handling of processed radiographs. Mount the radiographs promptly and enclose in protective envelope.

Inadequacies Attributable to Chemical Contamination

1. *White Spots on Film*
Probable cause: Premature contact with fixer—drops of fixer may have been splashed on workbench.
Correction: Clean workbench and place clean towel on work area before opening film packet.

2. *Dark Spots on Film* (Fig. 10-8)
Probable cause: Premature contact with developer—drops of developer
may have been splashed on workbench.
Correction: Clean workbench and place clean towel on work area before opening film packet.

3. *Iridescent Stain*
Probable cause: Oxidation and exhaustion of developer.
Correction: Replace the developer with fresh solution.

4. *Dark Brown or Gray Film*
Probable cause: Oxidation and exhaustion of fixer.
Correction: Replace the fixer with fresh solution.

5. *Brownish-Yellow Stains*
Probable cause: Insufficient or improper washing of the film.
Correction: Rinse in circulating cool water for at least 20 and preferably
30 minutes. Always return film that was taken out for "wet-reading"
for completion of fixing and washing.

inadequacies caused by fog on the film

Still another cause of inadequate radiographs is the formation of a
thin cloudy layer that fogs the film surface. Fog diminishes contrast
and makes it difficult and often impossible to interpret the radiograph. Fog on radiographs is produced in many ways and can occur
before or after the film is exposed or during processing. Most fogged
radiographs have a similar appearance and it is difficult to determine
the cause unless one knows, for example, that the film was outdated;
in that case one would suspect it to be age fog.

Fog Attributable to Causes During Storage

1. *Age Fog* (Fig. 10-9)
Probable cause: Overage film was used.
Correction: Watch date on film boxes. Use oldest film first.

2. *Chemical Fog*
Probable cause: Film stored in vicinity of fume producing chemicals.
Correction: Store film in cool, dry, fume-free area.

Fog Attributable to Causes Before or After Exposure

1. *Radiation Fog*
Probable cause: Film not properly protected before or after exposure.
Correction: Store film at safe distance from source of x-rays or protect
it by placing it in a lead-lined film dispenser. Never take more than one
film out of dispenser at a time and place film in film safe after exposure
is made.

Fog Attributable to Causes During Processing

1. *Safelight Fog*
Probable cause: Leaking safelight filter or prolonged exposure to safelight.
Correction: Check safelight for leaks. Minimize exposure to safelight.

2. *White Light Fog*
Probable cause: Light leak around door of darkroom or minute break in wrapping of the film.
Correction: Check darkroom for white light leaks. Avoid rough handling or bending of film packet.

3. *Processing Contamination Fog*
Probable cause: Contaminated processing chemicals.
Correction: Avoid contamination of processing chemicals. Always replace tank cover in the same way and rinse film to remove developer before moving the film hanger into the fixer insert.

conclusion

Faulty radiographs are traceable to many causes. Frequently several different errors may cause similar looking defects. A blank radiograph, for instance, may have been caused by failing to turn on the x-ray machine or by placing the exposed film into the fixer first. The auxiliary must learn which of these errors was most likely. Obviously, if the film is fresh, fog caused by aging is impossible, and if the processing chemicals have been changed recently, fog produced by exhaustion of the chemicals just can't happen. The well-trained auxiliary handles film carefully and develops neat work habits. The price of good diagnostic radiographs is expertise and meticulous attention to details in all stages.

bibliography

Ennis, Leroy M., Berry, Harrison M., and Phillips, James E. *Dental Roentgenology,* 6th ed. Philadelphia: Lea & Febiger, 1967.

O'Brien, Richard C. *Dental Radiography,* 2d ed. Philadelphia: W. B. Saunders Co., 1972.

Radiodontic Pitfalls, Rochester, N.Y.: Eastman Kodak Company, Radiography Markets Division, 1967.

Wilkins, Esther M. *Clinical Practice of the Dental Hygienist,* 3d ed. Philadelphia: Lea & Febiger, 1971.

Wuehrmann, Arthur H., and Manson-Hing, Lincoln R. *Dental Radiology,* 2d ed. St. Louis: The C. V. Mosby Co., 1969.

11

intraoral

radiographic procedures

intraoral procedures

Intraoral radiography consists of methods of exposing dental x-ray films within the oral cavity. It includes positioning the patient in the chair, selecting a film packet of suitable size, determining how the film is to be positioned and held in place while the exposure is made, aiming the PID, and setting the control devices correctly to make the exposure. All these steps need careful planning, because even a perfect radiograph is sometimes hard to interpret. Techniques described in this chapter will help the dental auxiliary make good radiographs.

There are three common types of intraoral examination. Each uses a slightly different film and technique, and each has a different objective. The first of these is the *periapical* examination, the fundamental purpose of which is to show the apices of the teeth and the structures that surround them. The second, the *interproximal* (bitewing) examination, is to show the coronal portions and the alveolar crests of both the maxillary and mandibular teeth of a given area on one film. The third type is the *occlusal* examination. Its purpose is to show the entire maxillary or mandibular arch (or a portion thereof) on a single film.

We have mentioned previously the two basic techniques employed in intraoral radiography—the *bisecting* and the *paralleling*. Either technique can be modified to meet special conditions and requirements. Each gives good results if one exercises care and remembers the fundamental principles of the technique. Each has advantages and limitations.

The first and earliest technique, still used by most, is called either the *bisecting,* the *bisecting-angle,* or the *short-cone* technique. The second and newer technique, now taught in most dental schools, is variously referred to as the *paralleling,* the *right-angle,* the *extension-cone,* or *long-cone* technique.

The majority of operators use the term "short-cone" for the bisecting and "long-cone" for the paralleling because the former uses a short cone or tube (PID) to establish an 8-inch target film distance whereas the latter uses a long PID to establish a target-film distance of 16 inches or more. Neither of these terms describes correctly the principles on which these techniques are based. The paralleling technique involves more than replacing the short PID with a longer one. As we have seen, the PID serves mainly to direct the central beam of radiation (central ray or CR) toward the teeth and the film. The terms "bisecting" and "paralleling" are more descriptive as these refer to the position in which the film is placed in relation to the teeth and to the direction from which the central beam passes through the teeth to the film to cast a shadow image. To avoid confusion, these techniques will be described as the bisecting and paralleling techniques in this text.

fundamentals of shadow casting

No matter which technique is used or how it is modified, the basic objective is to direct the PID toward the patient's face so that the central rays pass both horizontally and vertically through the tissues to be examined to the recording plane of the film at the most favorable angle. The film must be placed in relation to both the direction from which the x-ray photons originate (the source being on the target) and the intervening dental structures so that all parts of the resulting shadow image are shown on the radiograph with a minimum of distortion.

To understand the theory on which both intraoral techniques are based, remember the following: (1) the radiograph is a film with a shadow image; (2) the source of the x-ray photons is the focal spot on the target of the x-ray tube; and (3) the function of the film is to record the shadow image.

When a hand is placed between a nearby light source such as an electric bulb and a flat object such as a tabletop, the shadow of the hand becomes magnified and fuzzy when the distance between it and the tabletop is increased. The same happens in dental radiography where the tooth is the object and the film is the recording plane. To obtain a sharp and accurate shadow image, the two should be as close together as possible. The image can also be sharpened by increasing the distance between the light source and the object.

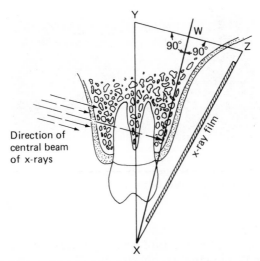

Fig. 11–1 Isometric triangle applied to the bisecting technique. Line XY passes through the long axis of a maxillary first premolar while film is positioned along line XZ. The central beam of radiation is directed perpendicularly through the apical area of the tooth toward the bisector XW. Since triangles WXY and WXZ are equal, the shadow image cast of the film will be approximately equal to the length of the film provided that the bisector line is correctly estimated. Most errors in foreshortening and elongation are traceable to incorrectly estimating the location of the bisector line.

Five basic rules for casting a shadow image apply whether the energy source is a light (as in photography) or x-ray photons (as in radiography): (1) The smallest possible source of light or radiation should be used; (2) the object and the recording plane should be as near to each other as possible; (3) the object and the recording plane should be parallel to each other; (4) the object should be as far as practical from the source; and (5) the light or radiation must strike both the object and the recording plane at right angles—in radiography, perpendicularly to the tooth and film.

Neither of the intraoral techniques completely meets these five requirements for accurate shadow casting. In the bisecting method the object and recording plane are not parallel to each other, and in the paralleling method the distance between the object and the recording plane is greater than ideal in most film placement areas.

principles of the bisecting technique

The concept of the bisecting technique originated in 1907 through the application of a geometric principle known as the "rule of isometry." This theorem states that two triangles having two equal angles and a common side are equal triangles (Fig. 11–1).

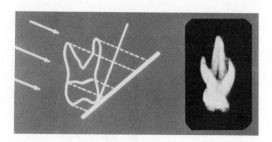

Fig. 11-2 Principle of the bisecting technique. The x-ray beam is directed per-
perpendicular to the imaginary lane that bisects the angle formed by the recording plane of the dental x-ray film and the long axis of the tooth. (Courtesy of
Rinn Corporation, Dental X-Ray Division.)

When this principle, known as Cieszynski's law, is applied to casting a shadow of a tooth on a film, the angle formed by the long axis
of the tooth and the plane of the film must be bisected and the beam
must be directed perpendicularly through the apex of the tooth
toward the bisecting line. One must first imagine a line, called the
bisector, and then direct the radiation beam to it instead of to the
long axis of the tooth or the film plane. This procedure is necessary
because the irregularities of the oral tissues and the curvature of the
palate seldom allow the film to lie parallel to the tooth when it is
held with the finger against the oral structures.

Theoretically, two isometric triangles (triangles having equal measurements) are formed when the central ray is directed perpendicularly
toward the bisector, and the film image that results should be the
same size as the tooth. However, in practice this does not always
happen. The image is usually satisfactory for diagnostic purposes,
but some dimensional distortion is inherent in the bisecting technique.

One of the disadvantages of the bisecting technique is that many
operators may have trouble estimating the direction of the bisector.
Thus, they may misdirect the central rays and cause the resulting
image to be either elongated or foreshortened. Another disadvantage
is that the divergence of the rays in the beam causes the image to appear slightly magnified. In order to cover the entire area of the film,
the rays have to diverge more when the target-object distance is short.
This divergence of the rays increases the closer the target is positioned
to the object; thus a degree of magnification is inevitable when an
8-inch target-film distance is used. Still another disadvantage is that
dimensional distortion occurs when the three-dimensional tooth and
bone structures are projected on the two-dimensional recording plane
of the film. This means that structures farther from the film will appear more elongated than those closer to the film (Fig. 11-2). Also

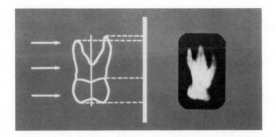

Fig. 11-3 Principle of the paralleling technique. The x-ray beam is directed perpendicular to the recording plane of the film which has been positioned parallel to the long axis of the tooth. (Courtesy of Rinn Corporation, Dental X-Ray Division.)

the steeper angle of vertical projection of the beam necessitated by directing the rays perpendicularly to the bisector instead of the tooth causes a shadow of the zygoma to be superimposed over the molar roots in the maxillary areas.

However, the bisecting technique does have advantages. Many believe it is the easier of the two methods to use. Moreover, the film can be held by finger pressure when a suitable film holder is not available. Although using a film holder is preferable to having the patient hold the film, the anatomical restrictions of the mouth or the patient's state of mind occasionally restrict its use. The bisecting method can be used in almost any situation.

principles of the paralleling technique

The paralleling technique was developed to solve some of the problems of the bisecting technique. In the paralleling technique the film is placed as nearly parallel to the long axes of the teeth as mouth anatomy permits. The central rays are directed at right angles [perpendiculary to both the teeth and film (Fig. 11-3)].

Normally, the target-film distance used in paralleling is 16 inches or longer. The accepted rule is that the distance between the target and the tooth should be as long as is practical and possible with the equipment used. It is also necessary to increase considerably the distance between the crowns of the teeth and the film. That is because oral structures, particularly the curvature of the palate, make it difficult to place the film with its recording plane parallel to the long axes of the teeth. One can only do this by using a film holder.

Once the technique is mastered, many find it just as easy as, if not easier than, the bisecting technique. Film placement is simpler and one need not locate the bisector. The paralleling technique was first developed by Franklin McCormack in 1920 and later improved and refined by Dr. Gordon Fitzgerald, Dr. William Updegrave, and many others.

Three things prevented rapid acceptance by the dental profession; the lack of x-ray machines that could operate at higher kilovoltages, the unavailability of high-speed films, and the absence of easy-to-use and accurate film holders.

As we said in Chapter 4, the beam of radiation diverges the farther it gets from its source and fans out like the spokes of a wheel. To prevent *adumbration* (the production of a fuzzy shadow around the outline of the image) and magnification of the image, the target-object distance must be as long as possible so that only the most central and parallel rays are directed at the tooth structures and film. The use of longer target-object distances diminishes the intensity of the radiation because the rays lose some of their energy as they travel through the air. Therefore, when greater velocity and penetrating power of the

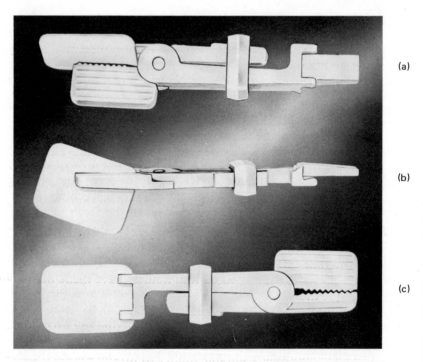

(a)

(b)

(c)

Fig. 11-4 The Rinn "Snap-a-Ray" film holder. This versatile film holder provides an excellent and simple method of standardizing the technique for intraoral radiography with the bisecting technique. The film is positioned to x-ray: (a) the anterior areas; (b) the mandibular third molar area; (c) the posterior areas. (Courtesy of Rinn Corporation, Dental X-Ray Division.)

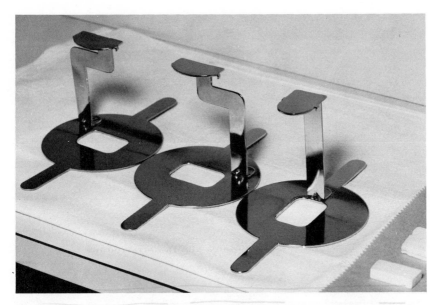

Fig. 11-5 Set of "Precision" child-adult instruments featuring metal collimating shield that restricts the x-ray beam to the size of the opening, providing just enough radiation to expose the film properly. (Courtesy of Precision X-Ray Company.)

rays is needed, greater kilovoltage is desirable. When the target-object distance is increased, the kilovoltage, milliamperage, exposure time, or a combination of these elements must be increased. The most common practice is to increase the exposure time by a factor of four when the target-object distance is doubled. Such prolonged exposures could not be safely and routinely made until films with very fast emulsion speed became available.

Films may be positioned in several ways. Biteblocks of various lengths can be used; the film can be fastened between two cotton rolls; or the film can be placed between the beaks of a hemostat. More advanced and sophisticated film holders have made the paralleling technique more common. The newest film holders vary from simple disposable biteblocks that require no sterilization to complex devices that indicate the correct angle for directing the PID in relation to the teeth and film (Figs. 11-4 through 11-6). Little trouble should arise in choosing a suitable holder to produce good results in most cases.

The only disadvantage of the paralleling technique is that it often takes more time to select, sterilize, and explain the purpose of a holder than simply to ask a patient to hold a film with a finger. This

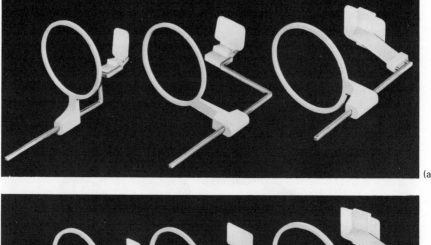

(a)

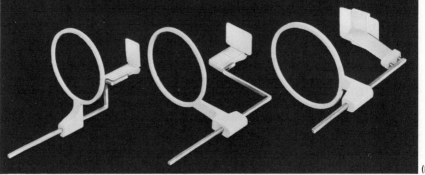

(b)

Fig. 11-6 Developed by Dr. William J. Updegrave, these two sets of film holders automatically indicate the correct horizontal and vertical angle, eliminating the need to numerically set the angulation and to place the patient's head in a predetermined position. The instruments shown are (a) The Rinn bisecting angle instruments used with the 8-inch target film distance; (b) the Rinn X-C-P instruments used with the 16-inch target film distance. On the left is the anterior instrument, in the center is the posterior instrument, and on the right is the interproximal (bitewing) instrument. Both sets of instruments are also available with rectangular placement holders. (Courtesy of Rinn Corporation, Dental X-Ray Division.)

is compensated for by the advantage that it takes less time to direct the rays perpendicular to the tooth than at a hard-to-locate bisector. A further advantage is that the image has only minimal dimensional distortion and magnification if care is applied in observing the rules of film positioning and aligning the film parallel with the teeth.

comparison of intraoral exposure techniques

As we have seen, both the bisecting and paralleling techniques are based on the rules of shadow casting. If the x-ray machine can gen-

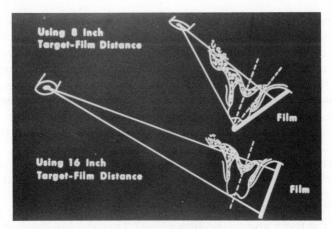

Fig. 11–7 Comparison of the bisecting and paralleling methods. In the bisecting angle method, the film is positioned adjacent to the tooth structure and the target film distance is approximately 8 inches, whereas in the paralleling method, the film is removed to near the center of the oral cavity where it must be retained in a position parallel to the long axes of the teeth and the target distance is approximately 16 inches. (Courtesy of Rinn Corporation, Dental X-Ray Division.)

erate sufficient milliamperage and kilovoltage, it can be used for either technique.

Proficiency should be developed in both techniques. Some offices have only one length PID and film holders available, or the dentist's preference may determine which technique must be used. Occasionally, technique modifications must be made. In some offices, for instance, the bisecting technique is used with the long PID. An operator using the paralleling technique may change to the bisecting method for one or two exposures during a full-mouth series because of anatomical limitations such as heavy muscle attachments or the shape of the palate.

The two techniques differ as to principles of shadow casting, procedures, and radiographic results.

Shadow Casting in the Two Techniques

Since most modern x-ray machines meet the requirements of either technique and the size of the effective focal spot is the same in both, the degree of adumbration or image distortion is affected by the distances and angles one selects (Fig. 11–7).

As we have seen, distances differ in the two techniques. The shorter 8-inch target-film distance is generally, but not necessarily, used in the bisecting method. In the paralleling method a 16-inch or longer distance is mandatory to minimize adumbration and magnification of the image. The use of a longer than conventional target-object distance in bisecting may improve the quality of the image slightly; however, a corresponding decrease of this distance in paralleling results in a very fuzzy image. With the exception of the mandibular molar areas, where film placement is almost identical with both techniques, a much shorter object-film distance is used in bisecting procedures. The film is placed as close to the teeth as possible, thus forming an angle between the long axes of the teeth and film. In paralleling procedures the film must be placed further from the teeth and parallel to them.

A further difference is in the angle at which the radiation strikes the tooth structures and the film plane. In the bisecting method the central rays are aimed perpendicularly to the bisector, while in the paralleling method they are directed perpendicularly to both the long axes of the teeth and to the film plane. Thus the bisecting method produces more dimensional distortion in most situations (Fig. 11–8).

Procedures for the Two Techniques

Procedures that differ for the two techniques include regulating the controls of the x-ray machine and determining the relationship between the position of the patient's head and the direction of the radiation beam. It should be remembered that the intensity of the radiation is diminished when the target-object distance is increased. To maintain intensity, corresponding increases must be made in milliamperage, kilovoltage, and exposure time. Although the amount of radiation that the patient receives is slightly less when the target-object distance is increased, the amount is insignificant.

Using the bisecting method, the patient may either hold the film with his finger or bite on a film holder; with the paralleling method,

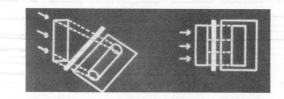

Fig. 11–8 The figure on the left shows dimensional distortion such as found in the bisecting technique. It occurs when a three-dimensional object is projected on a two-dimensional surface, creating an angular relationship between the object and the film. The part of the object farthest from the film is projected in an incorrect relationship to the parts closest to the film. Such distortion is eliminated in the paralleling technique, shown in the figure on the right. The film is positioned parallel to the object so that all parts of the object are in their true relationship to each other. (Courtesy of Rinn Corporation, Dental X-Ray Division.)

the patient must bite on a film holder. Unless special holders that indicate PID positions are used in the bisecting technique, the patient is usually seated upright with his head straight. This position is necessary for consistent results in determining the best horizontal and vertical angulations of the x-ray beam. Head positions and angulations are described in the next section. In the paralleling technique the patient's head can be in any position, so the patient can easily be placed horizontally in a contour chair. The horizontal angulation is determined in the same manner in both techniques. The vertical angulation necessarily differs because the rays are directed at the bisector instead of the long axes of the teeth.

Results with the Two Techniques

The final difference is in results. Reduced target-object distance means greater divergence between the rays and in the angle formed between the teeth and the film. Resulting images may not be anatomically accurate. Longer target-object distances and a more parallel relationship between the film and the tooth structures improve the quality of the radiographic image (Fig. 11–9).

horizontal and vertical angulation procedures

One of the most difficult procedures for the beginner to learn is how to determine the correct direction of the central beam in the horizontal and vertical planes.

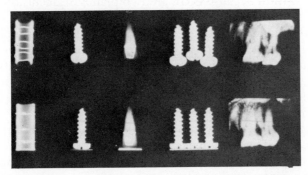

Fig. 11–9 The superior radiographic quality of the paralleling technique is readily demonstrated when results are compared. Radiographs produced by the bisecting technique (top) are not anatomically accurate in most instances, since obvious dimensional distortion is inherent in this technique. This kind of distortion does not occur with the paralleling technique (bottom) in which objects are reproduced in their normal size and relationship. (Courtesy of Rinn Corporation, Dental X-Ray Division.)

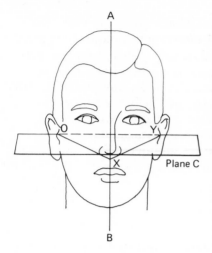

Fig. 11-10 Head divided by midsagittal plane A-B and occlusal plane C. The midsagittal plane must always be perpendicular to the floor and the occlusal plane must be parallel with the floor unless special film-holding devices, such as the Rinn bisecting-angle instruments, are used. The line O-X is the line of orientation for the maxillary teeth. It is also known as the *ala-tragus* line. The apices of the roots of the maxillary teeth are located close to this line. (From Ennis, Leroy M., et al. *Dental Roentgenology*, 6th ed. Philadelphia: Lea & Febiger, 1967.)

Although an experienced radiographer can expose radiographs with the patient either upright or prone, the use of predetermined head positions is recommended for the beginner. This makes it possible to standardize the procedure. With greater popularity of the contour chair, many are learning to make exposures with the patient in a prone position. The conventional position, particularly when bisecting, is to seat the patient upright and adjust the headrest so that the plane of occlusion for the jaw being examined is parallel to the plane of the floor, and the midsagittal plane that divides the patient's head into a right and left side is perpendicular to the plane of the floor (Fig. 11-10). This procedure requires periodic changes in the headrest position because there are two planes of occlusion when the mouth is open. One is the occlusal plane of the maxillary and the other of the mandibular teeth. The only time when both planes are the same is during the exposure of interproximal films, when the patient's mouth is closed as he bites on the bitetab. One must also realize that the occlusal plane is not a straight line but is usually curved. For this reason, the headrest position may have to be changed several times while making exposures on each jaw.

The angulation is changed by rotating the tube head horizontally and vertically. The x-ray machine is constructed with three swivel joints to support the yoke and tube head. One of these, located at the top and center of the yoke where it attaches to the extension arm, permits horizontal movement of the tube head to control the anteroposterior dimensions. The other two swivel joints are located at either side of the yoke. These permit the tube head to be rotated up or down in a vertical direction to control the longitudinal dimensions of the resulting image.

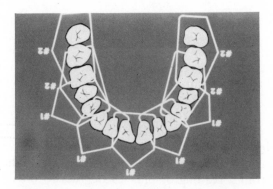

Fig. 11-11 The horizontal angulation is determined by directing the x-ray beam perpendicularly to the mean tangent of the teeth being radiographed, which is also the corresponding position of the film. The beam passes directly through the interproximal spaces. Standard #2 film is recommended in the posterior positions and narrow #1 film in the anterior areas. Horizontal angulation is determined in the same manner for the paralleling and bisecting technique. (Courtesy of Rinn Cor-Corporation, Dental X-Ray Division.)

The rules for determining the horizontal angulations were explained in the preceding sections. It should be remembered that the central rays are always directed perpendicularly to the mean tangent of the facial surfaces of the teeth and the film in both the bisecting and paralleling techniques (Fig. 11-11). As defined in this text, *horizontal angulation* is the direction of the central rays in a horizontal plane. To change their direction, one swivels the tube head from side to side. The best shadow image is obtained when the central rays can pass through the interproximal spaces. Deviation of the angulation toward the mesial or distal causes an overlapping of tooth shadows.

Rules for determining vertical angulations have also been explained. One must remember that in the bisecting technique the central rays are directed perpendicularly to the bisector, and in the paralleling technique toward the long axes of the teeth and the film. As defined in this text, *vertical angulation* is the direction of the central rays in a vertical plane. To change their direction, one turns the tube head on the yoke ends. Vertical angulation is customarily described in degrees. On most x-ray machines the vertical angles are scaled in intervals of 5 degrees on both sides of the yoke where the tube head is connected.

The vertical angulation of the tube head and the PID begins at zero. In that position the PID is parallel to the plane of the floor. All deviations from zero in which the tip of the PID is tilted toward the floor are called *positive* (plus) angulations. Those in which the PID is tipped upward toward the ceiling are called *negative* (minus) angulations.

The angulations just described are based on the assumption that the patient's midsagittal plane is perpendicular and that his occlusal plane is parallel to the plane of the floor. If the patient is positioned any other way—as for example, tilted back in the chair or with his head turned to either side—both the horizontal and the vertical angulations must be adjusted toward the long axes of the teeth and the occlusal plane instead of the plane of the floor. "Increasing or steepening" and "decreasing or flattening" are terms used to describe changes in degree of vertical angulation. For example, the positive angulation is increased by 20 degrees if the top of the PID is repositioned from a reading of plus 15 degrees to plus 35 degrees, and the negative angulation is decreased by 20 degrees if the tip of the PID is repositioned from a reading of minus 30 degrees to minus 10 degrees.

It is very easy, even when experienced, to err in estimating the location of the bisector or the long axes of the teeth. Such errors result in vertical distortion of the image. Many prefer to use film holders such as the X-C-P or the Bisecting-Angle Instruments (refer to Fig. 11–6) to reduce the chances for error. When the patient's head is in the conventional position, predetermined vertical angulations can be used in approximately 90 percent of all cases. Obviously, such angulations will vary from patient to patient. The average vertical angulations listed below are intended only as a guide and should not replace good judgment.

Maxillary incisors	——	plus 40 degrees
Maxillary canines	——	plus 45 degrees
Maxillary premolars	——	plus 30 degrees
Maxillary molars	——	plus 20 degrees
Mandibular molars	——	minus 5 degrees
Mandibular premolars	——	minus 10 degrees
Mandibular canines	——	minus 20 degrees
Mandibular incisors	——	minus 15 degrees

When the vault of the maxilla is flat or low, the average angulation should be increased by 5 to 10 degrees. It should be decreased by 5 to 10 degrees when the vault is high or steep. In the mandibular region, if the floor of the mouth is shallow or the teeth are facially inclined, the vertical angulation should be increased by 5 to 10 degrees. It should be decreased by 5 to 10 degrees when the floor of the mouth is very deep or the teeth incline lingually.

As already indicated, the degree of vertical angulation controls the longitudinal dimension of the image produced. When the vertical

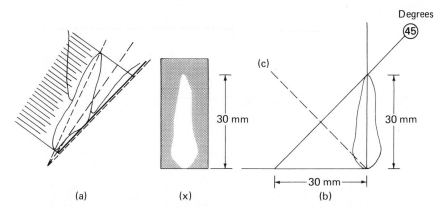

Fig. 11-12 (a) Rays directed perpendicular to the bisecting plane resulting in the correct projection of the tooth. (b) Tooth (33 mm in length) and the film forming an angle of 90 degrees. Rays were directed at 45 degrees (perpendicular to the bisecting plane (c), resulting in no distortion of the tooth, the result of which is shown in (x). (From Ennis, Leroy M. et al. *Dental Roentgenology*, 6th ed. Philadelphia: Lea & Febiger, 1967.)

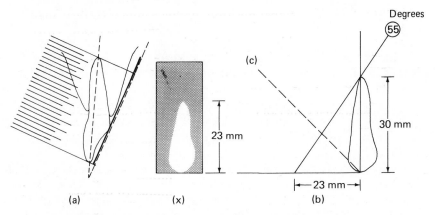

Fig. 11-13 (a) Rays directed perpendicular to the plane of the film resulting in a foreshortening of the root. (b) Tooth (30 mm in length) and film forming an angle of 90 degrees. Rays were directed at an angle of 55 degrees (plus 10 degrees) from a perpendicular to the bisecting plane (c), resulting in a 7 mm distortion (foreshortening) of the tooth, the result of which is shown in (x). (From Ennis, Leroy M. et al. *Dental Roentgenology*, 6th ed. Philadelphia: Lea & Febiger, 1967.)

angle is correctly estimated and the rays are directed perpendicularly to the bisector, no appreciable distortion results (Fig. 11-12). Excessive angulation, so that the direction of the rays is increased or steepened, foreshortens the image (Fig. 11-13). Insufficient angulation, so that the direction of the rays is decreased or flattened, elongates

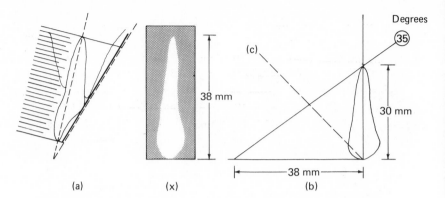

Fig. 11-14 (a) Rays directed perpendicular to the plane of the tooth resulting in longitudinal distortion of the root. (b) Tooth (30 mm in length) and film forming an angle of 90 degrees. Rays were directed at an angle of 35 degrees (minus 10 degrees) from a perpendicular to the bisecting plane (c), resulting in an 8 mm distortion (elongation) of the tooth, the result of which is shown in (x). (From Ennis, Leroy M. et al. *Dental Roentgenology*, 6th ed. Philadelphia: Lea & Febiger, 1967.)

the image (Fig. 11-14). It must always be considered that the tube head moves in both the horizontal and vertical planes. These movements must be coordinated if an accurate image is to be produced. It is seldom possible to position the tube head and PID correctly in both planes in one movement. The beginner, especially, should first determine the correct angulation in one plane and then in the other, being careful not to tilt the angulation that has already been established out of position. One should not make the exposure until satisfied that the angulation is properly coordinated in both planes in relation to the teeth and the film.

Chapter 9 referred to anatomic landmarks that can be used to determine the location of the apices of the teeth. When the patient is seated in the conventional position, the apices of the maxillary teeth are located along an imaginary line drawn from the ala of the nose to the tragus of the ear.

The following landmarks are helpful in determining the *point of entry* (the spot on the surface of the face at which the center of the tip of the PID and the central rays are directed). For maxillary teeth these are located along an extension of the ala-tragus line as follows: (1) the tip of the nose for the incisors, (2) the depression formed by the ala of the nose for the canines, (3) a point below the inner canthus of the eye for the premolars, and (4) a point below the outer canthus of the eye for the molars.

A point directly below the same landmarks and approximately 1/2 inch above an imaginary line from the symphysis of the chin to the tragus of the ear is used to locate the point of entry for the correspond-ing mandibular teeth. These points of entry are only approximations. In some cases, particularly where third molars are involved, these points are located farther distally. The truest image is produced when the central rays are directed through the point of entry toward the apices of the roots. However, the increased use of smaller beam diam-eters and film holders with collimating devices that limit the size of the beam makes it preferable to direct the central rays through the middle of the teeth instead of through the apices. The slightly elon-gated image that results does not lessen the diagnostic value of the radiograph.

preparing for radiographs

Unless the x-ray machine is located in the main operatory and the radiograph is to be exposed during dental procedures, advance prep-arations should be made. These save the time of both the patient and the operator.

First sanitize the entire area. Use a large piece of gauze moistened with alcohol or a disinfectant to wipe all parts of the machine that will be handled during the exposure—the yoke, the tube head, the PID, and the timer. Then turn on the x-ray machine and check that the dials work. If it is known in advance what technique will be used, attach the proper length PID and prepare film holders, if any. Always check the film dispenser to see if it contains an adequate supply of various sizes of films, including films with bitewing tabs.

Secure the patient's cooperation before any procedures are begun. New patients or young patients may be concerned with pain, and some patients are worried about safety. A few words of explanation will generally relieve the patient's anxiety. Explanations, of course, depend on the patient's understanding. As a rule, confidence will allay the patient's fears while hesitation increases them.

Whatever his understanding of radiation, the patient needs to know that modern equipment and high-speed films have reduced radiation exposures to safe levels and that radiographs are essential for making an adequate diagnosis. In simple language tell the patient how he benefits from the timely discovery of incipient decay, unsuspected impacted teeth, deep calculus formations, the location of unerupted teeth, and numerous other unsuspected conditions. An informed and cooperative patient always makes the task of producing good radiographs easier.

If the film is to be held by hand, explain how this should be done and ask the patient to wash his hands before sitting down in the dental chair. Eyeglasses and large earrings (which might get in the way of the PID) should be removed and put aside in a safe place. Check the mouth for dentures or removable bridgework. These should generally be removed because the clamps of partial dentures and removable bridges will be superimposed on the image of the teeth. Dentures, too, may be dislodged. The only time an appliance should be left in the mouth is when it is needed to stabilize the film holder or to bite on a tab.

After determining the age, general physique, and health of the patient, and completing the oral inspection for unusual conditions, one must decide whether the planned technique must be changed. During the oral examination observe (1) the position of the teeth, (2) the length of the crowns, (3) edentulous areas, (4) the thickness of the bone structures, (5) the general shape of the floor of the mouth and the palate, (6) the presence of lesions, unusual structures, loose teeth, or swelling, (7) the size of the tongue and oral opening, and (8) the flexibility of the lips and cheek muscles. On the basis of these observations, decide whether the patient is to hold the film with his finger or with a film holder. In selecting a holder, consider its weight, its ability to maintain the film in the proper position, its ease of use and sterilization, and the patient's comfort.

Adjust the headrest to whatever position the technique requires and drape the patient with a protective lead apron. Then show the patient how to hold the film, either with positive pressure of the thumb (maxillary areas) or index finger (mandibular areas) or with the film holder. Caution the patient to hold still while the exposure is made, so that the film will not be blurred or the relationship between film and the angulation of the PID lost.

Regulate the controls according to the technique and be sure that the patient knows what is expected of him before placing the film in the patient's mouth. Always position the film firmly and carefully; otherwise a gag reflex may begin. Gagging is a frequent problem and may be caused by apprehension or by a hypersensitivity of the oral tissues, particularly at the back of the mouth. One way to avoid or lessen gagging is to complete the exposure rapidly and remove the film immediately. Another is to premedicate the patient. This is extremely effective with children and extremely nervous patients. Still another method is to desensitize the nerve endings of the delicate mucosa by having the patient hold some ice water in his mouth for a short time before film placement or by spraying the sensitive areas with a topical anesthetic.

After each exposure, inspect the film for moisture and blot off excess saliva before placing the film in the film safe. After the final exposure, return all appliances, eyeglasses, and earrings to the patient. Lower the chair as far as it will go and give the patient an opportunity to wash his hands. Thank the patient for his cooperation and make an appointment for the diagnosis of his radiographs.

Final procedures include (1) identifying the films and removing them from the safe to the darkroom, (2) turning off the x-ray machine, and (3) sanitizing the room and equipment in preparation for the next patient.

bibliography

Ennis, Leroy M., Berry, Harrison M., and Phillips, James E. *Dental Roentgenology*, 6th ed. Philadelphia: Lea & Febiger, 1967.

O'Brien, Richard C. *Dental Radiography*, 2d ed. Philadelphia: W. B. Saunders Co., 1972.

Peterson, Shailer. *Clinical Dental Hygiene*, 3d ed. St. Louis: The C. V. Mosby Co., 1968.

Richardson, Richard E., and Barton, Roger E. *The Dental Assistant*, 4th ed. New York: McGraw-Hill Book Co., 1970.

Schwarzrock, Shirley Pratt, and Jensen, James R. *Effective Dental Assisting*, 4th ed. Dubuque, Iowa: William C. Brown Co., 1973.

Updegrave, William J. *New Horizons in Periapical and Interproximal Radiography*, Elgin, Ill.: Rinn Corporation, 1971.

Updegrave, William J. *Simplification and Standardization of the Bisecting-Angle and Interproximal Technics,* Elgin, Ill.: Rinn Corporation, 1971.

Wilkins, Esther M. *Clinical Practice of the Dental Hygienist*, 3d ed. Philadelphia: Lea & Febiger, 1971.

Wuehrmann, Arthur H., and Manson-Hing, Lincoln R. *Dental Radiology*, 2d ed. St. Louis: The C. V. Mosby Co., 1969.

X-Rays in Dentistry. Rochester, N.Y.: Eastman Kodak Co., 1972.

12

the periapical examination

film requirements for the periapical survey

A full-mouth series of periapical radiographs can provide the dentist with much valuable information about the patient's teeth and the bone structures that surround them. Individual radiographs focus attention on conditions that require treatment and serve as a guide in making the diagnosis and plan of treatment.

The periapical examination, frequently called the *full-mouth survey*, can be made with any of the four periapical film sizes (#00, #0, #1, #2) or any combination of these films. Film size depends upon (1) the age of the patient, (2) the size of the mouth opening, (3) the shape of the dental arches, (4) the presence or absence of unusual conditions or anatomical limitations, (5) the film holder and technique used, and (6) the patient's ability to tolerate the film. Normally, a minimum of fourteen films is used to cover the following tooth areas: (1) one film each for the maxillary and mandibular incisor area, (2) one film in each of the four canine (cuspid) areas (two in the maxillary and two in the mandibular arches), (3) one film in each of the four premolar (bicuspid) areas (two in the maxillary and two in the mandibular arches), and (4) one film in each of the molar areas (two in the maxillary and two in the mandibular arches). More films may be required for unusual conditions or for narrow arches requiring small films. The general rule is to use the largest film that can readily be positioned. Doing so keeps the number of exposures to a minimum.

Many dentists routinely prefer to use the narrow #1 intermediate film instead of the standard #2 film for exposures of the anterior teeth. Eight #1 films are generally used instead of six #2 films. Two

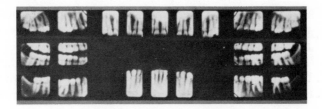

Fig. 12-1 The complete radiographic series shown includes four interproximal (bitewing) films in addition to the eight anterior and eight posterior periapical films. Although all of the exposures may be made with the standard #2 films when space permits, it is suggested that the narrow #1 film be used in all the anterior areas to assure patient comfort and easier placement without distortion. By using five narrow films in the maxillary anterior areas and three in the mandibular anterior areas, maximum accurate periapical and interproximal coverage can be obtained. (Courtesy of Rinn Corporation, Dental X-Ray Division.)

film combinations are often used when the narrow #1 film is employed: (1) five films for the maxillary anterior teeth—one each for the canines, one each for the laterals, and one film centered over the central incisors—and three films for the mandibular arch where the teeth are smaller—one film centered on each of the canines and the third film centered over the incisors; or (2) four films for the maxillary anterior teeth and four for the mandibular anterior teeth—the films centered over each of the canine and the central-lateral incisor regions.

Usually the standard #2 film is used to make the posterior periapical exposures. When space is limited, other film sizes may be used posteriorly (Fig. 12-1).

placement of the film packet

Regardless of which technique is used or how the film is held in place, correct placement of the film packet is important to prevent the film from bending or moving during exposure, thus causing distortion. Movement of the film, the patient, or the tube head will blur the radiograph or fail to show the intended teeth.

Warn the patient not to move during the exposure and make sure that the tube head stays put once it is in place. If it often moves or drifts after it is positioned, tighten the small wingnut on the tube arm. Watching the patient while getting ready to make the exposure is a cardinal rule. Particularly with the bisecting technique, when the PID is near the patient's nose, the patient may try to look at the rest of the tube head. In doing so he will tilt his head backward and move out of position. That movement elongates the teeth on the film.

With few exceptions, all films for the anterior areas are placed with the longest dimension of the film vertically and the films for the posterior areas are placed with the widest dimension horizontally. The edge of the film packet is placed parallel to, and protrudes 1/8 to 1/4 inch above or below the incisal or occlusal edges of the teeth.

One should develop a standard film placement for each region to be radiographed to insure that comparable serial radiographs can be made later. The tube side of the film is placed behind the teeth. Place films gently to prevent tissue irritation or gagging. Slight bending of the film corners toward the lingual makes it easier to place the film and increases the patient's comfort. However, excessive bending of the film results in creases, streaks, and distortion.

Most film manufacturers show the location of the identification dot by a small circle or dot on the *back side* of the film. Film mounting is easier if the identification dot is always positioned toward the occlusal or incisal edges.

It is always best to keep the film surface as flat as possible. A film holder with a backing plate on the biteblock makes this almost automatic. However, when the film is held by finger pressure, some additional support may be needed to keep it from bending in the middle. One means of support is to insert one or two cotton rolls between the film packet and the lingual surfaces of the teeth. Such a technique is particularly effective in the anterior regions and when the mandible has very sharp curvature. Besides minimizing film bending, the use of cotton rolls between teeth and film may produce a more parallel relationship and increase patient comfort.

sequence of film positioning

Opinions differ as to which region should be exposed first in making a full-mouth survey. Some operators prefer to make the first exposure in the right maxillary region and continue in sequence to the left maxillary molar region, then drop down to the left mandibular molar region, finishing in the right mandibular molar region. Others prefer a similar sequence but with the directions reversed, while still others begin with the mandibular anterior exposures, on the theory that the patient is less liable to gag when a film is placed in this region than when it is placed in the upper molar region where the tissues are more sensitive. Gagging is frequently psychological. If the first few films produce no discomfort, the patient will become used to the feel of the film in his mouth and accept it.

With an experienced operator who can place the film skillfully and rapidly, it probably makes very little difference which area is exposed first. But the same system of film placement should always be followed to make sure that all regions are exposed.

film retention for bisecting procedures

However the film is held, both vertical and horizontal angulations are dependent on specific positions of the patient's head and correct film placement. Unfortunately, perfect results are very difficult to achieve because placement, head alignment, and angulations are matters of judgment and subject to errors. Several sophisticated film holders have been developed to overcome such variables. Among these are the Anterior Bisecting-Angle Instrument (Fig. 12-2) and the Posterior Bisecting-Angle Instrument (Fig. 12-3). These instruments are easy to assemble, position in the mouth, and sterilize. In most cases they are far superior to having the patient hold the film. These instruments can be used with any PID. However, they are generally most effectively used with a short open-cone type or the new rectangular collimated type.

When correctly used, these instruments reduce errors of judgment by automatically indicating correct horizontal and vertical angulation.

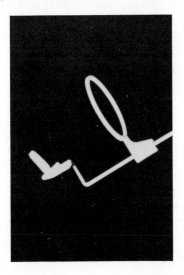

Fig. 12-2 Assembled Rinn anterior bisecting-angle instrument. Consists of a metal indicator rod offset for use in both maxillary and mandibular anterior areas, a plastic locator ring, and a plastic bite block with a backing plate tilted at an average angle to place the film close to the lingual anatomy. To assemble, hold the offset portion of the stainless steel indicator rod (arm) away from the biting surface of the block, insert the pins of the rod into the receptacle holes in the bite block, and slide the plastic locator ring opposite the bite block. The use of the narrow #1 film is suggested. This film is inserted vertically into the block and rests against the backing plate. The anterior instrument is also available with a rectangular film placement holder for use instead of the circular locator ring. (Courtesy of Rinn Corporation, Dental X-Ray Division.)

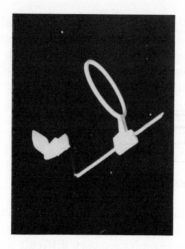

Fig. 12-3 Assembled Rinn posterior bisecting-angle instrument. Consists of right angle metal indicator rod, offset plastic locator ring, and plastic posterior bite block with tilted backing plate. The instrument is assembled in a similar manner to the anterior instrument. When thus assembled, the instrument can be used for either maxillary right and mandibular left or vice versa. Position of bite block and locator ring must be reversed on the indicator rod when changing to the opposite areas. The standard #2 film is positioned horizontally in the bite block. The instrument can also be used with a rectangular placement holder having alignment studs to fit into collimated rectangular PID. (Courtesy of Rinn Corporation, Dental X-Ray Division.)

Thus they eliminate the need to set the angulations numerically or to place the patient's head in a predetermined position. They also simplify and standardize the technique, making duplication of postoperative radiographs easier. They also minimize curved film plane distortion and eliminate cone cutting. Because many offices do not have such instruments, the technique described in the next section is based on finger-held film.

mandibular periapical exposures: bisecting technique

The *mandibular incisor* region is shown in Figure 12-4. If the #2 film is used, it is centered at the midline and all four incisors will be shown on the radiograph. Number 1 film may either be centered at the midline or to the right or left of the midline so that the center of the film is between the central and lateral incisors. To make this exposure, the following steps are suggested:

1.   Seat the patient in the conventional position and adjust the headrest so that the sagittal plane of the head is perpendicular to the plane of the floor. Use the tragus to corner of the mouth line as a guide, so that the incisal plane of the anterior teeth is also parallel with the plane of the floor.

2.   Grasp the film at its narrow edge between the index finger and thumb. Insert the film vertically with the tube side of the film toward the teeth. Center the film over the area of interest, either at the midline or between the central and lateral incisor. Direct the lower edge of the film toward the floor of the mouth. Use the index finger of the opposite hand to guide the film as close to the lingual surfaces of the

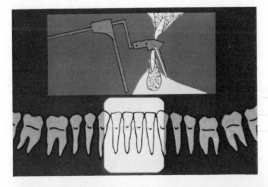
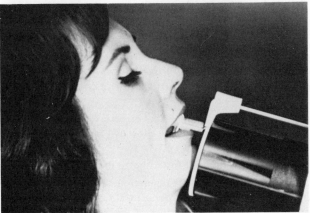

(a)

(b)

Fig. 12-4 The mandibular incisor area. (a) Diagram showing positioning of x-ray film using the bisecting-angle instrument. To insert the film packet, grasp it between thumb and finger and place the shielded (printed) side of the film packet against the backing support of the bite block and insert vertically into the slot. In this illustration, a standard #2 film is shown. Generally the use of narrow #1 film is preferred. (b) Photograph showing position of bisecting-angle instrument and short open-ended cone type PID with patient. (Courtesy of Rinn Corporation, Dental X-Ray Division.)

teeth as possible. If resistance is encountered, ask the patient to first raise and then relax his tongue. In cases of extreme curvature of the mandible, bend the film slightly toward the lingual in the two lower film corners.

3.   Place the film with its upper edge parallel toward the incisal edges of the teeth and protruding about 1/4 inch above them. For uniformity of appearance in mounting, position all periapical films with the identification mark toward the incisal or occlusal edge.

4.   Instruct the patient to hold the film with the index finger of either hand by exerting a slight pressure against the upper middle of the film. A cotton roll may be placed between the film and the tooth to avoid

bending the film and shaping it to the arch. Ask the patient to raise his elbow so that it is level with his shoulder and place his thumb under the mandible to brace it against movement.

5.   Establish the vertical angulation by determining the location of the bisector (half way between the long axis of the tooth and the film plane). In most instances this will be between minus 15 and minus 20 degrees.

6.   Establish the horizontal angulation by directing the central rays through the embrasures either between the central incisors or between the central and lateral incisors perpendicularly toward the film.

7.   Center the PID over the point of entry, a point on the chin about an inch above the lower border of the mandible. Adjust the tip of the PID so that it almost touches against the skin.

8.   Make the exposure. Follow film manufacturer's suggestions to determine optimal milliamperage, kilovoltage, and exposure time.

To make exposures in the *manbidular canine* (cuspid) region, follow the same basic procedures but make the following changes:

1.   Place the film as for the preceding exposure, but center it vertically over the canine and first premolar. Allow 1/4 inch to protrude over the incisal edges.

2.   Place the anterior border of the film to include the lateral incisor.

3.   Slightly increase the vertical angulation, usually to between minus 20 and minus 25 degrees. Direct the central rays perpendicularly toward the mean tangent of the labial surface of the canine. The point of entry is near the center of the root of the canine, about an inch above the inferior border of the mandible.

4.   Make the exposure according to film manufacturer's directions.

To make exposures in the *mandibular premolar* (bicuspid) region, follow the same basic procedures but make the following changes (Fig. 12-5):

1.   Place the film as before with minor modifications. Grasp the film at the corner and insert it with the widest dimension horizontally. Use the index finger of the opposite hand to press the film against the lingual. Center the film over the premolar area and move the film forward enough so that the front edge covers the distal of the canine. Allow about 1/8 inch of the film to protrude above the occlusal surfaces of the teeth.

2.   Change the vertical angulation as needed, usually between minus 10 to minus 15 degrees, and direct the central rays horizontally to pass through the embrasure between the second premolar and the first molar.

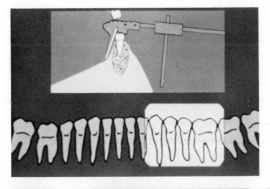

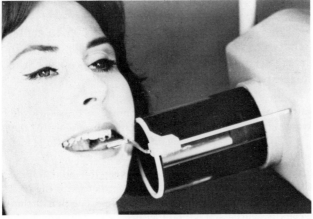

(a)

(b)

Fig. 12-5 The mandibular premolar area. (a) Diagram showing the positioning of the x-ray film and the bisecting-angle instrument. Film is placed with widest dimension horizontally in the bite block and centered over the second mandibular premolar. Relief or slight rolling of the edge of the anterior, inferior corner of the film packet will facilitate positioning. (b) Photograph of patient showing position of bisecting-angle instrument and short open-ended PID. (Courtesy of Rinn Corporation, Dental X-Ray Division.)

The point of entry is near a point below the pupil of the eye and about 1/2 inch above the lower border of the mandible.

3. Make the exposure according to the film manufacturer's directions.

To make an exposure in the *mandibular molar* region, follow the same basic procedures but with the following changes:

1. Make adjustments in the occlusal plane because this often curves in the molar area. Place the film in the same manner as before but center the film between the first and second molar. Unless the main interest is in the third molar area, place the film forward enough to cover the distal of the second premolar.

2.   Decrease the vertical angle as indicated by position of the bisector, usually minus 5 to minus 10 degrees, and direct the central rays horizontally to pass through the embrasure between the first and second molar. The point of entry is near a point below the outer canthus of the eye and about 1/2 inch above the lower border of the mandible (further back for third molar exposures).

3.   Make the exposures according to the film manufacturer's directions.

maxillary periapical exposures: bisecting technique

The *maxillary incisor* region. If the #2 film is used, it is centered at the midline and both central and lateral incisors are shown on the same film. If the exposure is made with the narrower #1 film, less of the lateral incisors will be shown. Many prefer to center the narrower film between the central and lateral incisors. This requires a film for the right and left side. To make this exposure, the following steps are suggested:

1.   Seat the patient in the conventional position and adjust the head-rest so that the sagittal plane of the head is perpendicular to the plane of the floor. Use the tragus-to-ala line as a guide so that the incisal plane of the anterior teeth is parallel with the plane of the floor.

2.   Grasp the film at its narrow edge between the index finger and thumb and insert it vertically with the tube side toward the teeth and palate. Center the film over the area of interest, either at the midline or between the central and lateral incisors. Direct the upper edge of the film toward the palate. Use the index finger of the opposite hand to guide the film toward the palate. It is often advisable to place a cotton roll between the film and the teeth to prevent bending the film. Make sure that the film margin is even with the edges of the teeth and allow about 1/8 inch of the film to protrude below the edges.

3.   Instruct the patient to hold the film with the thumb by exerting a slight pressure against the lower middle part of the film. Either thumb may be used if the film is centered at midline, otherwise ask him to use the hand opposite to the side on which the film is placed. Ask the patient to raise his elbow and rest the other fingers against the face to prevent movement of the film.

4.   Establish the vertical angulation by determining the location of the bisector. In most instances this will be between plus 40 and plus 45 degrees.

5.   Establish the horizontal angulation by directing the central rays through the embrasure either between the central incisors or between the central and lateral incisors perpendicularly toward the film.

6.   Center the PID over the point of entry near the tip of the nose. Adjust the PID so that its tip almost touches the patient's skin.

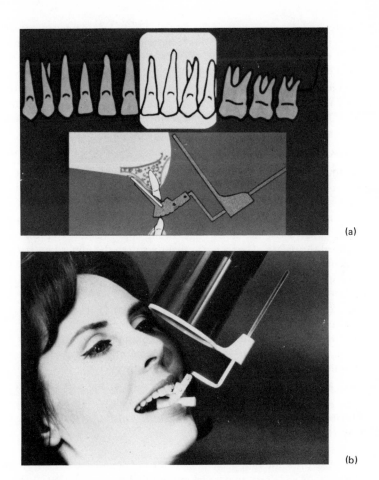

(a)

(b)

Fig. 12-6 The maxillary canine (cuspid) area. (a) Diagram showing the position of the x-ray film and the bisecting-angle instrument. Film is centered vertically in the bite block over the canine (cuspid) area and positioned against the lingual surface as close as anatomy will permit. Standard #2 film is shown. However, #1 film is suggested. (b) Photograph of patient showing position of bisecting-angle instrument and short open-type PID. (Courtesy of Rinn Corporation, Dental X-Ray Division.)

7. Make the exposure. Follow the film manufacturer's suggestions to determine optimal milliamperage, kilovoltage, and exposure time.

To make the exposure of the *maxillary canine* (cuspid) region (Fig. 12-6), follow these steps:

1. Use essentially the same procedures for film placement as for the central incisors. Position the film vertically so that the canine is in the

center and the distal part of the lateral is included. Allow an incisal margin of about 1/8 inch. On rare occasions place the film diagonally over the canine.

2.   Slightly increase the vertical angulation, usually to between plus 45 and plus 50 degrees. Direct the central rays perpendicularly toward the mean tangent of the labial surface of the canine. The point of entry is near the center of the root of the canine, at the ala of the nose.

3.   Make the exposure according to the film manufacturer's directions.

To make exposures in the *maxillary premolar* region, follow the same basic procedures but make these changes:

1.   Grasp the film at the corner and insert it with the widest dimension horizontally. Use the index finger of the opposite hand to press the film toward the palate. If necessary, slightly soften the upper film corners to conform with the shape of the palate. Center the film over the premolar area and position it so the distal half of the canine is included. Allow a 1/8 inch occlusal margin.

2.   Change the vertical angulation as needed, usually to between plus 30 and plus 35 degrees, and direct the central rays to pass through the embrasure between the first and second premolar perpendicularly to the film. Direct the center of the PID to the point of entry, located on the tragus-ala line directly below the pupil of the eye.

3.   Make the exposure according to the film manufacturer's directions.

To make an exposure of the *maxillary molar* region (Fig. 12-7), follow these steps:

1.   Use the same film placement as for the premolars, but adjust the headrest as necessary to parallel the occlusal plane with that of the floor. Center the film over the molar area and let the front edge of the film cover the distal half of the second premolar. Occasionally, it may be desirable to position the film further back to include erupting third molars.

2.   Change the vertical angulation as needed, usually to between plus 20 and plus 25 degrees. Depending on whether third molars are impacted or not, the vertical angulation required may be as steep as plus 55 degrees. Direct the central rays horizontally through the embrasure between the first and second molar perpendicularly toward the film. The point of entry is on the tragus-ala line, directly below the outer canthus of the eye. When unerupted or impacted third molars are suspected, direct the center of the PID about 1/2 inch further back and higher.

3.   Make the exposure according to the film manufacturer's directions.

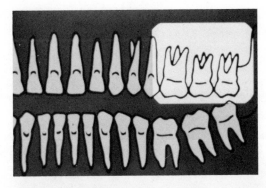

(a)

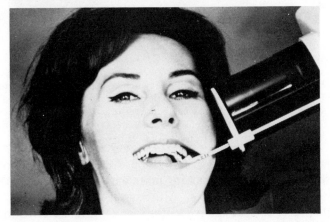

(b)

Fig. 12–7 The maxillary molar area. (a) Diagram showing position of x-ray film with widest dimension placed horizontally. In the maxillary molar area, the posterior block is positioned on occlusal surface with anterior border of the film aligned with anterior surface of first molar and as close to the lingual surface as anatomy permits. (b) Photograph of patient showing position of bisecting-angle instrument and short circular open-type PID. (Courtesy of Rinn Corporation, Dental X-Ray Division.)

film retention for paralleling procedures

As previously indicated, a film holder is needed with the paralleling technique. Simplest are wood, plastic, or styrofoam biteblocks with a backing plate and slot for film retention. The film can be inserted either vertically for the anteriors or horizontally for the posteriors. The same biteblock can be used on all exposures. Slightly more complex is the Snap-A-Ray Holder, a double-ended instrument which holds the film between two plastic jaws that are locked in place. The

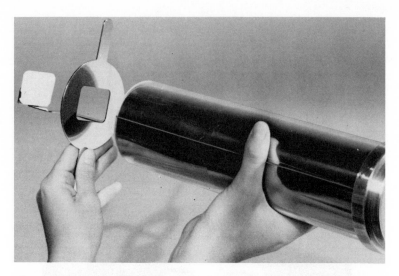

Fig. 12-8 Metal "Precision" posterior x-ray film holder for use with long round metal-type PID. The metal collimating shield, combined with the lead-lined cone restrict the size of the x-ray beam and reduce tissue radiation. Precision instruments are available for anterior, posterior, and interproximal radiography in adult and child sizes. (Courtesy of Precision X-Ray Company.)

plastic jaw serves as a bite plane in the posterior areas. The other end of the instrument is a backing plate with a slot which holds the film during anterior exposures. Although it is not necessary, most operators prefer to seat the patient upright in the conventional manner when simple blocks or the Snap-A-Ray is used. More complex still are the metal Precision film holders (Fig. 12-8) which have a metal facial shield attached to an arm on which the patient bites. At the end of the arm a backing plate supports the film and holds it parallel to the shield. The X-C-P (Extension Cone Paralleling) instruments (Fig. 12-9) and the rectangular collimated X-C-P instruments (Fig. 12-10) function in a similar manner. The more complex instruments must be assembled prior to use and have separate components for anterior and posterior positioning. Both the Precision and the X-C-P instruments were developed in an attempt to simplify paralleling procedures and minimize dimensional distortion. These instruments are easy to sterilize, simple to position, and highly adaptable in that the patient may be in any position.

The X-C-P instruments, designed by Dr. Updegrave, consist of an anterior and posterior instrument. Each instrument, like the Bisecting-Angle instruments that have been described earlier, consists of a plastic biteblock, a metal indicator rod with which the PID is aligned in a parallel manner, and a locator ring which allows the operator to line

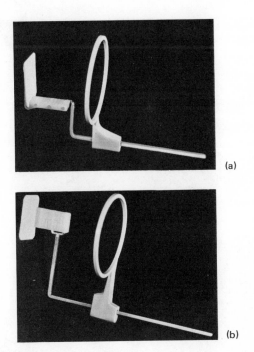

(a)

(b)

Fig. 12-9 The Rinn X-C-P instruments shown here are assembled in the same manner as the bisecting-angle instruments, the only difference being in the bite block and that they are intended for use with the 16-inch target-film distance. The backing plate of the X-C-P bite blocks are at right angles to the biting plane to hold the film parallel to the teeth instead of being tilted at an average angle as in bisecting. (a) The Anterior X-C-P instrument fully assembled with film positioned vertically. (b) The Posterior X-C-P instrument fully assembled with film positioned horizontally. (Courtesy of Rinn Corporation, Dental X-Ray Division.)

up the PID with it and thus direct the central beam directly at the middle of the film. One can use either the circular locator ring with the long circular open extension tube or the rectangular holder with the open rectangular PID.

Because it is not practical to describe the technique for the use of each of the many available film holders, the descriptions and illustrations for the following sequence of tooth regions is based on the use of the X-C-P instruments. Other instruments require slight changes in technique.

mandibular periapical exposures: paralleling technique

To make an exposure of the *mandibular incisor* region, follow these steps:

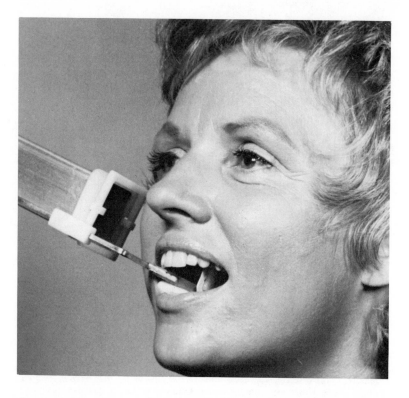

Fig. 12–10 Rectangular instrumentation for reduced tissue exposure. Lead-lined rectangular PID limits the size of x-ray beam. Slots on the PID align with studs on the placement holder. Both the X-C-P and the bisecting-angle instruments can be modified by substituting the rectangular placement holder for the circular indicator ring and changing to a long or short rectangular PID. The use of the lead-lined collimating device makes possible reductions of 50 percent or more in tissue exposure area. (Courtesy of Rinn Corporation, Dental X-Ray Division.)

1.   Place the patient's head in any comfortable position within convenient reach of the PID.

2.   Insert the film vertically into the slot of the film holder with the tube side of the film toward the lingual of the teeth.

3.   Insert the film and holder by directing the lower edge of the film toward the floor of the mouth and against the frenum of the tongue. Do this by first turning the film holder so that the film is parallel with the floor and then gradually raising the holder so that the film assumes a vertical position in the mouth. If resistance is encountered, ask the patient to first raise and then relax his tongue.

4.   Push the film holder back far enough to achieve parallelism and center the film on the midline or between central and lateral incisors if right and left exposures are to be made. Although the #2 film is occasionally used, the narrow #1 film is preferred for all anterior exposures.

Place a cotton roll between the biteblock and the maxillary teeth and ask the patient to close firmly on the block.

5.   Slide the locator ring to about 1/2 inch from the skin surface and align the PID with the rod and ring on vertical and horizontal planes. If anatomical restrictions in the mouth make it impossible to parallel the film with the long axes of the teeth or if the variance in the angle between teeth and film appears to be greater than 15 degrees, establish the vertical and horizontal angulations in the same way as when using the bisecting technique.

6.   Make the exposure according to the film manufacturer's directions. Remember that the paralleling technique uses double the target-film distance of the bisecting technique. Thus, according to the inverse square law, the exposure time must be quadrupled to achieve the same degree of film density when milliamperage and kilovoltage are not changed.

To make an exposure of the *mandibular canine* (cuspid) region, follow these steps:

1.   Use the same film placement procedure as for the mandibular incisor but center the film over the canine.

2.   Instruct the patient to close on the block and slide the locator ring to near the skin surface. Align the PID with both rod and ring on horizontal and vertical planes.

3.   Make the exposure according to film manufacturer's directions.

To make an exposure of the *mandibular premolar* (bicuspid) region (Fig. 12-11), follow these steps:

1.   Follow the same basic procedures as for the canine exposure but use the larger #2 film and place it with its widest dimension horizontally. If the teeth are too long to show the root apices, place the film vertically. This is seldom necessary.

2.   Position the film in the mouth centered over the second premolar. (Soften the lower front corner of the film if necessary for easier placement.)

3.   Instruct the patient to close on the block and slide the locator ring to about 1/2 inch from the skin. Align the PID with both rod and ring on horizontal and vertical planes.

4.   Make the exposure according to the film manufacturer's directions.

To make an exposure of the *mandibular molar* regions, follow these steps:

1.   Use the same placement procedures as for the mandibular premolar regions but place the anterior film border to include the distal of the second premolar. The center of the film is between the first and second

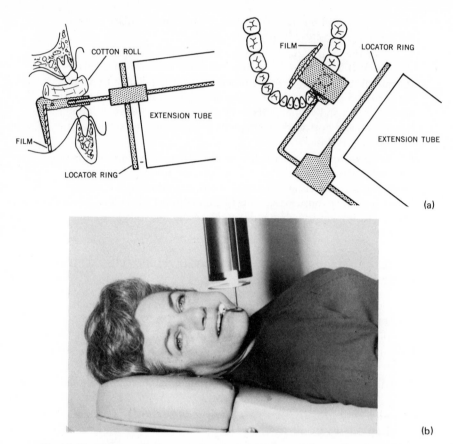

Fig. 12-11 The mandibular premolar area. (a) Diagrams show relationship of film, teeth, X-C-P instrument, and extension tube (PID length required for 16-inch T/F distance). Film is positioned with widest dimension horizontally in posterior areas and parallel to teeth, further toward lingual area than in bisecting technique. A cotton roll should always be between the opposing teeth and the bite block, causing the opposing teeth to force the bite block firmly against the biting surfaces of the teeth to be x-rayed. In cases of short teeth, it may be advisable to insert a second cotton roll between the block and the mandibular teeth to raise the film and prevent unnecessary impingement of the film on the floor of the mouth. (b) Photograph showing patient in supine position. With both the bisecting-angle and the X-C-P instruments, the necessity of definite head positioning with respect to occlusal and sagittal alignment is eliminated, regardless of the type of chair employed. (Courtesy of Rinn Corporation, Dental X-Ray Division.)

molars. In this region the film slides into the sulcus between the teeth and the tongue and close to the teeth.

2.   Instruct the patient to close on the block and slide the locator ring to about 1/2 inch from the skin surface. Align the PID with both rod and ring on horizontal and vertical planes.

3.   Make the exposure according to film manufacturer's directions.

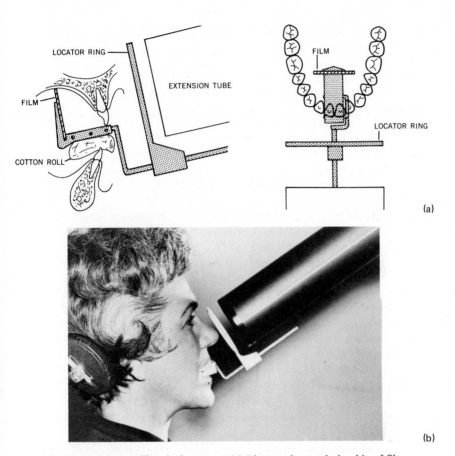

LOCATOR RING

EXTENSION TUBE

FILM

COTTON ROLL

FILM

LOCATOR RING

(a)

(b)

Fig. 12-12 The maxillary incisor area. (a) Diagram shows relationship of film, teeth, X-C-P instrument, and extension tube (long PID). As in all anterior areas, film is positioned with longest dimension vertically. Film is parallel to teeth with the block inserted to its full length to position the film back toward the region of the first molars (in the posterior areas, the film packet is placed back toward the midline of the palate) to obtain adequate space. Failure to push the film far enough lingually results in an impingement of the film on the curvature of the palate which in turn results in an absence of apical structures and excessive occlusal margin. (b) Photograph of patient showing position of X-C-P instrument and long circular open-type PID. (Courtesy of Rinn Corporation, Dental X-Ray Division.)

maxillary periapical exposures: paralleling technique

To make an exposure of the *maxillary incisor* region (Fig. 12–12), use the following steps:

1.   Place the patient's head in any comfortable position within convenient reach of the PID.

2.   Insert the film vertically into the slot of the film holder with the tube side of the film toward the lingual of the teeth.

3.   Insert the biteblock far enough into the mouth (about 1 inch) so that the upper edge of the film contacts the palate in the first molar area and is parallel to the labial planes of the incisors. Depending on the number of films to be exposed in the incisor area, center the film at the midline or between the central and lateral incisors.

4.   Rest the biteblock on the incisal edges and insert a cotton roll between the block and the mandibular teeth. Ask the patient to close firmly.

5.   Slide the locator ring down the indicator rod to about 1/2 inch from the skin and align the PID with both rod and ring on vertical and horizontal planes.

6.   Make the exposure according to the film manufacturer's directions.

For the *maxillary canine* (cuspid) region, follow these steps:

1.   Use the same film placement as for the incisors, with some minor changes. Center the film over the canine and include the distal of the lateral incisor.

2.   Instruct the patient to close on the block and slide the locator ring down the indicator rod to about 1/2 inch from the skin. Align the PID with both rod and ring on horizontal and vertical planes.

3.   Make the exposure according to film manufacturer's directions.

For the *maxillary premolar* (bicuspid) region, follow these steps:

1.   Follow the same basic procedures as for the canine exposure but use the larger #2 film and place it with its widest dimension horizontally. Insert the biteblock far enough into the mouth so that the upper edge of the film contacts the palate near the midline. Softening the upper front corner of the film makes positioning easier. Center the film over the second premolar so that the anterior border of the film covers the distal portion of the canine.

2.   Instruct the patient to close on the block and slide the locator ring down the indicator rod to about 1/2 inch from the skin. Align the PID with both rod and ring on horizontal and vertical planes.

3.   Make the exposure according to the film manufacturer's instructions.

For the *maxillary molar* region, use the following steps:

1.   Use film placement very similar to that for the premolar region. Center the film over the embrasure between the first and second molars

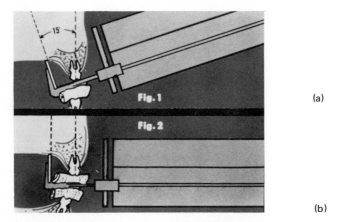

(a)

(b)

Fig. 12-13 Maxillary molar variations. Absolute parallelism between the film
and the long axes of the teeth in patients with low palatal vaults. (a) If the discrepancy does not exceed 15 degrees, usually the resulting radiograph is acceptable. (b) By using two cotton rolls, one on each side of the block, the film can
be paralleled with the long axes. However, the area of periapical coverage will
be reduced. This is often adequate, particularly if the teeth have short roots.
Greater periapical coverage can be obtained if the vertical angulation of the PID
is increased by 5 to 15 degrees over what the instrument indicates. (Courtesy of
Rinn Corporation, Dental X-Ray Division.)

and so that the anterior film border covers the distal portion of the second premolar. Place the film further to the back if the center of interest
is the third molar.

2.   Instruct the patient to close on the block and slide the locator ring
down the indicator rod to about 1/2 inch from the skin. Align the PID
with both the rod and ring on horizontal and vertical planes.

3.   Make the exposure according to the film manufacturer's instructions.

maxillary molar variations

Because of anatomic limitations, rotation of the teeth, variations
in the height of the palate, the presence of unerupted third molars,
or excessive root lengths, one must occasionally depart from the
usual procedures. Such changes include horizontal or vertical angulation, and film placement.

1.   Frequently the embrasures between the molars are not at right
angles to the plane of a film that is parallel to the mean tangent of the
buccal surfaces of the teeth. Consequently, overlapping of the contact
areas results. One can overcome this by a slight alteration of the film
placement so that the anterior border of the film is further toward the
lingual than the posterior.

2.   Occasionally, radiographs exposed in the conventional position show the buccal roots superimposed over the lingual roots so that a correct diagnosis is impossible. One can often correct this by altering the relationship of the film to the teeth in the horizontal plane. Here it may be necessary to place the anterior border of the film close to and the posterior border toward the lingual and farther away from the teeth.

3.   Often a conventionally positioned film that shows the tuberosity region reveals a coronal portion of a third molar to be at the level of apices of the second molar. In this case, one places the film as far back as anatomy and patient-comfort permit. Drastic changes in both vertical and horizontal angulations may be required. This varies according to the location of the imbedded tooth.

4.   Absolute parallelism between the film and the long axes of the teeth is difficult to accomplish in patients with low palatal vaults. If the discrepancy from parallelism does not exceed 15 percent, the radiograph is generally acceptable. In many instances, one can solve the problem of low vault by using two cotton rolls, one on each side of the block. These may parallel the film with the long axes adequately, but will reduce periapical coverage. Occasionally, especially when the roots are longer than average, one can increase periapical coverage by making the vertical angulation 5 to 15 degrees greater than indicated (Fig. 12–13).

conclusion

Bone and tissue density vary with the age and physical structure of the patient. Moreover, in most persons the bone structures are thinnest in the mandibular incisor region and densest in the maxillary molar region. Thus, for the best radiographs, it is often desirable to deviate slightly from the film manufacturer's suggestions and make minor changes in milliamperage to vary the film density, changes in kilovoltage to alter the contrast, or to make changes in the exposure time. However, many operators prefer a given exposure time for a film of a given sensitivity (film speed), slightly increasing it for the maxillary molars and decreasing it for the mandibular incisors. Obviously, exposure time must be decreased for children and edentulous patients. As experience is gained, most operators learn to make variations based on age, size, estimated density of the bone structures.

bibliography

Ennis, Leroy M., Berry, Harrison M., and Phillips, James E. *Dental Roentgenology,* 6th ed. Philadelphia: Lea & Febiger, 1967.

O'Brien, Richard C. *Dental Radiography,* 2d ed. Philadelphia: W. B. Saunders Co., 1972.

Peterson, Shailer. *Clinical Dental Hygiene,* 3d ed. St. Louis: The C. V. Mosby Co., 1968.

Richardson, Richard E., and Barton, Roger E. *The Dental Assistant,* 4th ed. New York: McGraw-Hill Book Co., 1970.

Updegrave, William J. *New Horizons in Periapical and Interproximal Radiography,* Elgin, Ill.: Rinn Corporation, 1971.

Updegrave, William J. *Simplification and Standardization of the Bisecting-Angle and Interproximal Technics,* Elgin, Ill.: Rinn Corporation, 1971.

Wainwright, William Ward. *Dental Radiology,* New York: McGraw-Hill Book Co., 1965.

Weissman, Donald D., and Longhurst, Gerald E. *Manual of Rectangular Field Collimation for Intraoral Periapical Radiography,* Los Angeles: UCLA Press, 1971.

Wilkins, Esther M. *Clinical Practice of the Dental Hygienist,* 3d ed. Philadelphia: Lea & Febiger, 1971.

Wuehrmann, Arthur H., and Manson-Hing, Lincoln R. *Dental Radiology,* 2d ed. St. Louis: The C. V. Mosby Co., 1969.

X-Rays in Dentistry, Rochester, N.Y.: Eastman Kodak Co., 1972.

13

interproximal

or bitewing examination

fundamentals of interproximal radiography

The interproximal or bitewing examination is made either in conjunction with the complete periapical examination (usually repeated at intervals of from two to six years) or alone at the time of the six-month or annual regular inspection.

Because dental caries frequently begin in the interproximal areas of the teeth and periodontal disturbances near the gingival line, most operative and preventive treatment is performed in this part of the dental arches. Thus, interproximal radiographs that show the crowns and alveolar crests of both the maxillary and mandibular teeth on the same film are ideal for identifying these problems.

An advantage of the interproximal over the periapical film is that it can be positioned near and almost parallel to the teeth of both arches when the patient's jaws are firmly closed. This often makes it possible to see decay and the height of the alveolar crests better than on periapical films of the same area because the film is closer to the teeth and the central ray can be directed at a more ideal angle than is possible in bisecting. One of the great values of the interproximal radiograph is that it reveals caries in the earliest stages. This is particularly important in the premolar and molar regions, where small carious lesions are often concealed by the wide buccolingual diameters of these teeth. Such lesions are frequently unnoticed in a visual inspection. A disadvantage of the interproximal radiograph is that it does not show apical conditions or lesions.

The interproximal exposure can be made with either the short or long PID because both the bisecting and paralleling principles are combined in this technique. The film is positioned almost parallel to the long axes of the teeth and the divergence of the vertical angulation is so slight that the final result is about the same as is obtained when the paralleling technique is used. In fact, many dentists who use the paralleling technique routinely do not include interproximal radiographs with the complete periapical survey because the same structures are shown in the same way. However, this is only true if ideal angulation is achieved when the periapical films are exposed. Thus, it is still a good idea to supplement the periapical survey with interproximal radiographs.

However, interproximal radiographs should always supplement a full-mouth periapical survey made with the bisecting technique, because the latter uses a much greater vertical angle for projecting the central rays than is generally necessary when paralleling. The steeper angle may distort the shape of the lesion or project it so that it is hidden behind a metal restoration, thus not accurately showing the location or size of the decayed area.

The interproximal survey can be made with two to eight films, using any size from #00 through #3, or any combination of these. Exposures can be made in both the anterior and posterior areas of the mouth. Anterior exposures are rarely made because they seldom show anything not shown on properly positioned periapical films. Moreover, caries are much easier to detect by digital examination and strong transillumination in the anterior than in the posterior teeth.

Because over 95 percent of all interproximal exposures are made in the posterior (premolar and molar) regions, the manufacturers package most film sizes with bitetabs attached to them. If such special films are not stocked in the office, it is easy to paste a bitetab to the tube side of the selected periapical film or to slide the film into a bite loop, thus converting it into an interproximal film. For posterior use, fasten the tab or slide the film into the loop so that the film can be positioned in the mouth with its longest dimension horizontally.

The length and curvature of the posterior arches vary in all individuals. A single small film placed in each arch often provides adequate coverage for all areas of interest in a small child or young adult. On most adults, four #2 films (two on each side) are generally preferred; however, some dentists routinely make the posterior survey with one #3 (extra-long) film on each side. When compared with the standard #2 film, the longer film has two serious disadvantages. One is that in most dental arches there are two slightly divergent pathways of the posterior teeth, one for the premolars and the other for the molars. As the central rays pass through these divergent embrasures, the interproximal structures overlap on the radiograph. The other is that the long film is too narrow to reveal all of the periodontal bone level.

The horizontal angulation for interproximal exposures is the same as that used for periapical ones of the same area. The vertical angulation is a compromise between that used in the bisecting technique for the maxillary and mandibular areas. Generally, plus 10 degrees for the anterior areas and plus 8 degrees for the posterior areas is used. For example, if plus 40 degrees is used for the maxillary central incisors and minus 20 degrees for the mandibular central incisors, the spread is 60 degrees. Half of this, subtracted from plus 40 degrees or added to minus 20 degrees, gives a compromise angulation of plus 10 degrees. By the same logic, if plus 20 degrees is used for the maxillary molar and minus 5 degrees is used for the mandibular molar, the compromise angulation is about plus 8 degrees.

The point of entry for the central beam for all interproximal exposures is on the level of the incisal or occlusal plane (near the lip line) at a point opposite the center of the film.

methods of holding the interproximal film packet in position

Several methods are used to stabilize the film; all of them make use of some type of bitetab, film loop, or biteblock. Because anterior films must be placed vertically in the mouth, bitetabs which can be fastened to the tube side with adhesive are easiest to use. The film loop, into which the film can be slid with the tube side facing the tab, and bite planes are most often used for posterior exposures. In offices where more exacting techniques are employed, periapical films are used with metal or plastic film holders. One such holder is the metal bitewing instrument (Fig. 13-1), in child or adult size. A hard paper film loop into which the film is placed so that the exposure side faces the lingual of the teeth is attached to two wire prongs. The patient bites on a plastic block which is fastened to the biting plane of the instrument. The patient closes on the block and supports the instrument with his hand while the PID is positioned flush with the collimator plate during the exposure.

Another film holder is the combination metal and plastic interproximal instrument (Fig. 13-2). This instrument is similar in appearance to the Bisecting-Angle and X-C-P instruments described in Chapter 12. It differs in that the indicator rod is straight and short and that the plastic block has two slots between which the film is inserted with the exposure side (tube side) facing the thin biting plane of the block.

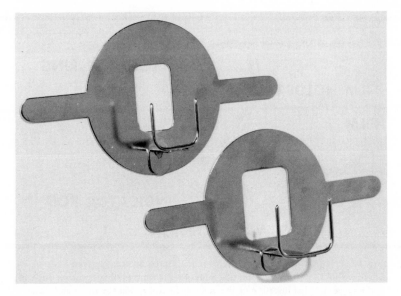

Fig. 13-1 Child and adult "Precision" bitewing (interproximal) instrument. A special paper double bitewing loop holds the film in place. One end of the double loop fits over the U-shaped wire and the film packet is held by the loop at the other end. (Courtesy of Precision X-Ray Company.)

Either the conventional round locator ring or the newer rectangular placement holder can be used with the long or short PID to align the central beam vertically and horizontally at the most advantageous angle.

The metal or metal and plastic film holders are easy to sterilize, assemble, and position. By eliminating the necessity for numerical angulation or specific head positioning, many of the common errors such as cone cutting, closed interproximal spaces, overlapping crowns, and diagonal occlusal planes can be reduced when film holders are used. Specific instructions are available from the various manufacturers. The exposure techniques that follow are based on the use of bitetabs or film loops as the more complex film holders are not available in many offices. Because the overwhelming majority of interproximal films are exposed in the premolar and molar regions, the techniques for the posterior exposures is described first.

posterior interproximal exposures

Unless special film holders are used, it is generally best to seat the patient upright in the conventional position. Three major film packet positions are generally preferred. If two exposures are to be made on

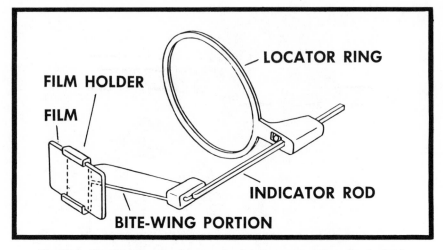

Fig. 13-2 The Rinn bitewing (interproximal) instrument consists of a plastic bite block with a thin biting portion that supports the film-holding device at one end and a receptacle for insertion of the metal indicator rod at the other end. A locator ring slides over the rod. The instrument is also available with a rectangular film-placement holder for use with the collimated rectangular PID. (Courtesy of Rinn Corporation, Dental X-Ray Division.)

each side, position one film in the molar and the other in the premolar region. Otherwise center a single film between the molars and premolars (Fig. 13-3). Although vertical angulations may vary slightly from patient to patient, the average vertical angulation used is plus 8 degrees. Regardless of technique used, the horizontal angulation is directed perpendicularly through the embrasures toward the film.

To make the *molar interproximal* exposure, follow these steps:

1. Position the patient comfortably and adjust the headrest so that the midsagittal plane of his head is perpendicular and the occlusal plane parallel with that of the floor.

2. Attach a bitetab or slip the film into a loop if special film is not available. The standard #2 film is generally most satisfactory. If necessary, slightly soften the film corners to conform to the curvature of the arch.

3. Grasp the tab and position the lower half of the film so that it is centered over the mandibular second molar. Cover the distal part of the second premolar with the front edge of the film.

4. Hold the tab firmly against the occlusal surface of the mandibular teeth. Ask the patient to close his mouth so that the teeth occlude normally. Biting down correctly on the tab is important to obtain proper relationship of the teeth on the radiograph. Sometimes, practice without the film will help patients understand how to bite. Failure

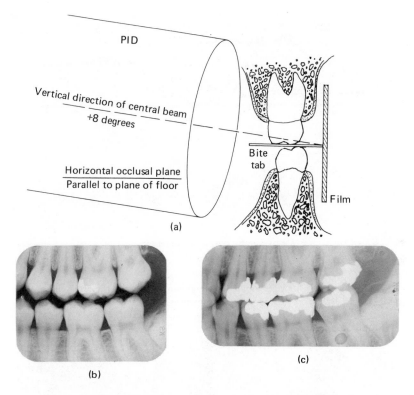

(a)

(b)

(c)

Fig. 13-3 Posterior interproximal area.   (a) Film slips into loop with widest dimension parallel to occlusal plane. Film packet is stabilized by bite tab that rests on the occlusal surfaces of the mandibular teeth. Patient closes on tab to immobilize the film.   PID is projected vertically at +8 degrees toward center of film and the central beam is directed horizontally through the interproximal spaces. Any size film packet from #00 through #3 may be used.   (b) Radiograph of molar interproximal area made with standard #2 film.   (c) Radiograph of pre-molar-molar area made with the long #3 film.

to hold the tab firmly permits the film to drift lingually and increases the possibility that the tongue will move the film. This often results in a slanted occlusal plane. Caution patient to bite firmly.

5.   Center the PID over the point of entry—a spot on the occlusal plane between the maxillary and mandibular first molars. Establish the vertical angulation, usually at plus 8 degrees, and direct the horizontal angulation through the mean tangent of the embrasures perpendicularly toward the recording plane of the film.

6.   Make the exposures according to the film manufacturer's directions.

The *premolar interproximal* exposure is practically identical to the one described for the molars, with these exceptions:

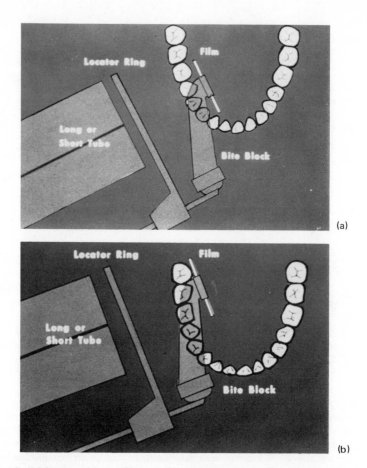

Fig. 13-4 Diagrams showing film and PID position with the Rinn bitewing (interproximal) instrument: (a) Premolar position made in conventional manner; (b) recommended molar position. Since the interproximal surfaces of the molar teeth are in a mesio-distal relationship to the sagittal plane, conventional positioning of the film parallel to the sagittal plane or to the buccal surfaces will result in overlapping of the contact areas and closure of the embrasure spaces. To avoid this distortion, it is recommended that the film be positioned perpendicular to the embrasures, resulting in a diagonal placement of the film, with the anterior border at a greater distance from the lingual surface of the teeth than the posterior border. (Courtesy of Rinn Corporation, Dental X-Ray Division.)

1.   Adjust the occlusal plane if necessary. Center the film over the second mandibular premolar. Cover the distal of the mandibular canine with front of film.

2.   Center the PID over the point of entry—a spot on the occlusal plane between the maxillary and mandibular second premolars.

The *premolar-molar interproximal* exposure is also identical to the exposures described, with these exceptions:

1. Unless the arch is extremely short, use the long #3 film and center it over the embrasure between the mandibular second premolar and first molar.

2. Attempt to direct the central rays perpendicularly at the mean tangents of the interproximal spaces of both the premolars and molars. This is not always possible, particularly if the arch curves, and overlapping in the proximal areas may result. That is why it is generally better to expose the premolar and molar areas separately.

Because the interproximal surfaces of the molars are in a mesiodistal relationship to the patient's sagittal plane, conventional film placement parallel to the buccal surfaces often results in overlapping of the contact areas and closure of the embrasure spaces. In such cases, position the film perpendicularly to the embrasures to avoid this distortion. Place the film slightly diagonally with the front edge of the film further from the lingual of the teeth than the back part (Fig. 13–4).

anterior interproximal exposures

When making anterior interproximal exposures seat the patient in the same position and establish the horizontal angulation in the same manner as for the posterior exposures. Increase the vertical angulation to plus 10 degrees. For ease of placement and least distortion, use the narrow #1 films. Since these exposures are seldom made, special film holders are not available. Use a longer bitetab (about 1 inch long) than is used for the posterior exposures and attach it to the tube side in such a manner that the film can be placed in the mouth with its longest dimension vertically. This allows the film to be placed further lingually in the mouth and prevents bending of the film in the middle as the tab is pulled forward when the patient is asked to bite with the teeth in edge-to-edge position on the tab.

To make an exposure of the *incisor interproximal* area (Fig. 13–5), follow these steps:

1. Position the patient comfortably and adjust the headrest so that the midsagittal plane of his head is perpendicular and the incisal plane is parallel with that of the floor.

2. Slightly soften all four corners of the film for greater patient comfort. Grasp the bitetab and position the lower half of the film so that it

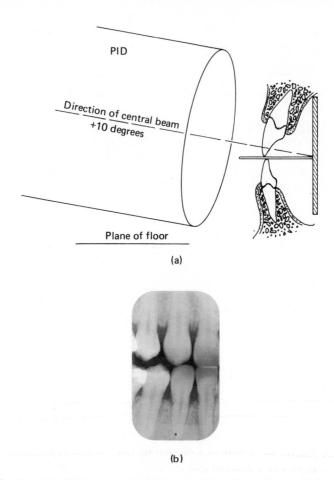

Fig. 13–5 Anterior interproximal area. (a) Center film packet vertically at mid-line and stabilize by patient gently closing on tab at incisal edges of teeth. Teeth meet tab in end to end position. Suggested vertical angulation is +10 degrees toward the center of the film and horizontally the x-ray beam is directed through the interproximal spaces. (b) Interproximal film of the canine area.

is either centered at the midline, or if two films are to be used, between the central and lateral incisors. Direct the lower edge of the film into the space between the teeth and tongue.

3. Hold the bitetab so that it rests on the incisal edge of the mandibular incisor and ask the patient to close gently but firmly on it in an edge-to-edge position. Push the upper part of the film toward the lingual if it appears to prematurely come into contact with the palate. Exert only a gentle pull forward on the tab—just enough to take up any slack and prevent the film from turning.

4. Center the PID over the point of entry—a spot at the incisal line between the maxillary and mandibular incisors. Direct the vertical an-

gulation at about plus 10 degrees. Establish the horizontal angulation by directing the central rays perpendicularly through the mean tangent of the embrasures between either the central incisors or between the central and lateral incisors toward the plane of the film.

5.   Make the exposure according to the film manufacturer's directions.

To make the *canine interproximal* exposure, follow the same procedures as for the incisor area but center the film over the canine, with the front edge of the film including the distal of the mandibular laterial incisor. The point of entry is opposite the maxillary canine at the incisal edge.

bibliography

Ennis, Leroy M., Berry, Harrison M., and Phillips, James E. *Dental Roentgenology,* 6th ed. Philadelphia: Lea & Febiger, 1967.

O'Brien, Richard C. *Dental Radiography*, 2d ed. Philadelphia: W. B. Saunders Co., 1972.

Peterson, Shailer. *Clinical Dental Hygiene*, 3d ed. St. Louis: The C. V. Mosby Co., 1968.

Updegrave, William J. *New Horizons in Periapical and Interproximal Radiography*, Elgin, Ill.: Rinn Corporation, 1971.

Updegrave, William J. *Simplification and Standardization of the Bisecting-Angle and Interproximal Technics,* Elgin, Ill.: Rinn Corporation, 1971.

Wilkins, Esther M. *Clinical Practice of the Dental Hygienist*, 3d ed. Philadelphia: Lea & Febiger, 1971.

Wuehrmann, Arthur H., and Manson-Hing, Lincoln R. *Dental Radiology*, 2d ed. St. Louis: The C. V. Mosby Co., 1969.

X-Rays in Dentistry, Rochester, N.Y.: Eastman Kodak Co., 1972.

14

the occlusal examination

reasons for making the occlusal examination

The occlusal examination may be made alone or to supplement periapical or interproximal radiographs. The large #4 occlusal film is very useful for recording information that cannot be adequately recorded on the smaller periapical films—for example, whole lesions. If the patient can open his mouth enough for the occlusal film, such film can show the total extent of a maxillary fracture.

In addition to locating fractures, the occlusal film can be used to make a rapid survey of the mouth to locate impacted or supernumerary teeth; foreign bodies; cysts (sac or capsule containing a liquid or semisolid substance); odontomas (tumors derived from tissues involved in tooth formation); osteomyelitis (an inflammation of the bone); and malignancies. It can also measure changes in size and shape of the dental arches; reveal the presence of stones blocking the passage of Wharton's duct (exit to the submaxillary gland) in the floor of the mouth; indicate the size and shape of tori on the mandible; show the progress of healing in the maxillae following a cleft palate operation; locate retained roots, unerupted teeth or foreign particles on edentulous arches; and do many other special things.

Although an occlusal film may sometimes not provide as complete and satisfactory information as a periapical film, the occlusal film can be used when it is desirable to view the area of interest in its entirety or when placement of periapical films is too difficult. For example, a patient with swollen cheeks may be unable to open his mouth wide enough. A young child may misunderstand instructions for holding the film in place or may have oral tissues that are so sensitive that he cannot tolerate periapical film. Most children can cooperate in biting on a film, and smaller films than the occlusal should be used for them.

technical considerations

In addition to the large occlusal film generally used to make the occlusal survey, smaller intraoral films may also be used, depending on the area to be examined. The standard #2 periapical film is frequently used with children, either to make a rapid survey of labiolingual or buccolingual unerupted tooth positions or in place of periapical positioning. It is also used on adults when the mouth is too small for the large occlusal film. A variety of film positions can be used to make the occlusal examination. The film may be placed with its longest dimension either parallel or at right angles to the patient's midsagittal plane. It may also be centered over one small sector, over the anterior portion of the arch, or over the entire right or left dental arch. Placement and size of film depend on the information needed.

Most occlusal film packets contain two films. When they do, both films can be developed alike to give duplicate films. If duplicate films are not needed, one film can be developed fully for 4½ minutes at 68° F. while the other film is developed for only 2½ minutes. The fully developed film will show all details of the hard structures, whereas the underdeveloped film will show the soft structures.

Any occlusal exposure can be made with the short or long PID. However, the occlusal technique is based on the correlation of certain head positions with specific vertical angulations. Most occlusal exposures are made with the patient's midsagittal plane perpendicular to the plane of the floor. When maxillary exposures are made, the occlusal plane of the teeth is parallel to the plane of the floor; however, when the mandibular exposures are made, the patient is reclined in the chair and the occlusal plane may be perpendicular to the plane of the floor. Regardless of how the patient is positioned, the *tube side* of the film must always face toward the occlusal surfaces of the teeth in the arch being examined. The film is held in place during the exposure by slight pressure of the teeth of the opposite jaw. When the arches are edentulous, the patient holds the film with his thumbs.

Occlusal films may be either topographical or cross-sectional. When exposing an occlusal film topographically (Fig. 14–1), the rules of bisecting are followed and the radiation is directed through the apices of the teeth perpendicularly toward the bisector. Because a larger area is involved and it is not always possible to use the most favorable

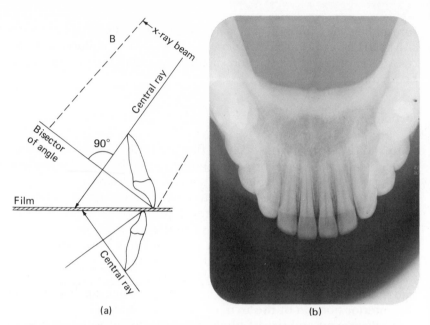

(a)   (b)

Fig. 14-1 (a) Diagram illustrating angulation theory of topographic projections. A topographical radiograph appears similar to ordinary periapical film except that it is larger. The exposure side of the film is placed toward the teeth to be examined in such a way that the shadow of the questionable area will be cast onto the film when the exposure is made. A similar procedure is used for film placement for posterior areas except that the film is positioned more distally toward the side being examined. Angulation rules for topographical projections are identical to those for the bisecting technique. Using either short or long PID, the radiation is directed through the apex of the teeth at right angles to the bisector. Vertical angulations are increased when examining areas in the distal part of the palate. (b) A typical radiograph of a mandibular anterior exposure. (From Wuehrmann, Arthur H., and Manson-Hing, Lincoln R. *Dental Radiology*, 2d ed. St. Louis: The C. V. Mosby Co., 1969.)

vertical angle, the images of the teeth generally appear longer than on periapical radiographs.

The patient's head position and film position may be identical for making a topographical or cross-sectional exposure. The difference is in the direction of the central ray. In the cross-sectional technique, the central ray is directed toward the area of interest and *parallel* with the long axes of the teeth and adjacent areas. This results in a circular or elliptical appearance of the teeth on the radiograph (Fig. 14-2).

Film placement, angulation, and exposure procedures vary with the location and type of condition. Only a few simple, common techniques are described in this chapter.

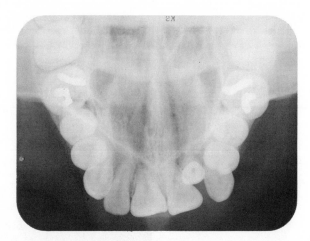

Fig. 14-2 Typical radiograph of a maxillary cross-section view. Such a view can be made of a specific area or of the entire dental arch. The film is placed in the same manner as for the topographical view, but the central beam of radiation is directed toward the area of interest parallel to the long axis of the teeth included in the area of interest or directly adjacent to it. The teeth appear as round or elliptical areas on the film. When it is desired to observe the entire arch, the central beam is directed perpendicular to the film.

the maxillary occlusal examination

The Maxillary Incisor Survey (Fig. 14-3)

The following sequence of steps is suggested to make this exposure:

1. Seat the patient and adjust the headrest so that the midsagittal plane is perpendicular and the occlusal plane of the maxillary teeth is parallel to the plane of the floor.

2. Insert the film between the occlusal surfaces of the teeth with the tube side toward the palate and the longest dimension of the film parallel to the midsagittal plane.

3. Ease the film into the mouth until it contacts the tissues that cover the anterior borders of the rami of the mandible. An alternate method is to slide the film slightly to either side to obtain an oblique view of the teeth.

4. Instruct the patient to close gently but firmly with his teeth against the film to immobilize it.

5. Establish the horizontal angulation so that the central ray is parallel with the patient's midsagittal plane, and set the vertical angulation at about plus 65 degrees to the plane of occlusion.

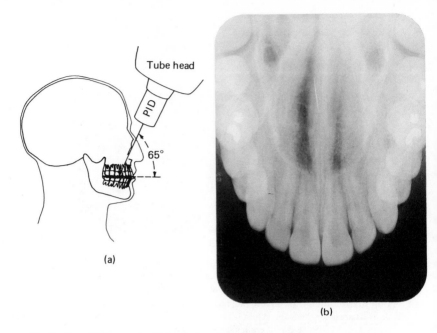

(a)

(b)

Fig. 14-3 (a) Diagram showing relationship of tube head and PID to occlusal film and patient for a topographical view of the maxillary incisor area. Exposure side of film faces maxillary arch with longest film dimension antero-posteriorly. Horizontal central beam is parallel with patient's midsagittal plane and the vertical angulation is approximately +65 degrees through a point near the bridge of the nose. The radiation beam is directed toward the center of the film. Slight modifications in film placement and angulation can be made when the center of interest is in the canine or molar area or when a cross-sectional view is desired. (b) Typical radiograph of topographical maxillary incisor area.

6.   Direct the PID toward the center of the film through the point of entry. On adults, this is the bridge of the nose and on children the tip of the nose.

7.   Set the timer, adjust controls as warranted, and make the exposure.

The Modified Maxillary Arch Survey

Follow the same procedure as was suggested for the maxillary incisor survey with these exceptions:

1.   Insert the film in the mouth with the longest dimension at right angles with the midsagittal plane.

2.   Establish the horizontal angulation at 0 degrees to the midsagittal plane and set the vertical angulation at about plus 75 degrees to the plane of occlusion.

3.   Direct the PID toward the center of the film through the point of
entry near the bulge of the nose.
4.   Set the timer, adjust the controls as warranted, and make the exposure.

The maxillary incisor technique can be modified for exposures of
the canine, molar, or sinus areas by making slight changes in film
placement and the central ray angulations. To make the canine survey, shift the film laterally to either the right or left side. Direct the
central ray horizontally at about 45 degrees to the midsagittal plane,
and vertically at about plus 60 degrees. The point of entry is in the
canine fossa, at a point near the infraorbital foramen. The film is
shifted laterally in the same manner to make the molar survey. Use
the same vertical angulation but change the horizontal angulation so
it is at 90 degrees to the midsagittal plane. The point of entry is immediately below the outer canthus of the eye. To obtain a sinus
survey, establish the horizontal angulation at 0 degrees to the midsagittal plane, and set the vertical angulation at plus 80 degrees. Direct
the central ray toward the center of the film through a point of entry
in the canine fossa. In this procedure the maxillary sinus is directly
above the film. This exposure is occasionally made to locate root
tips in the sinus.
If the maxillary arch is edentulous, position the film with its longest
dimension at right angles with the midsagittal plane. The patient
presses the film against the ridge with his thumbs and braces his other
fingers against the side of the face to prevent the film from moving.
If the patient has a lower denture, it may be left in the mouth to bite
against the film.

the mandibular occlusal examination

The Mandibular Incisor Survey

The following sequence of steps is suggested to make this exposure:

1.   Seat the patient and adjust the headrest so that the midsagittal
plane is perpendicular and the plane of occlusion is at a 45-degree angle
to the plane of the floor.
2.   Insert the film between the occlusal surfaces of the teeth with the
tube side toward the floor of the mouth and the longest dimension of
the film parallel to the midsagittal plane.
3.   Ease the film into the mouth until the rear edge of the film touches
the tissues covering the front borders of the rami of the mandible. An

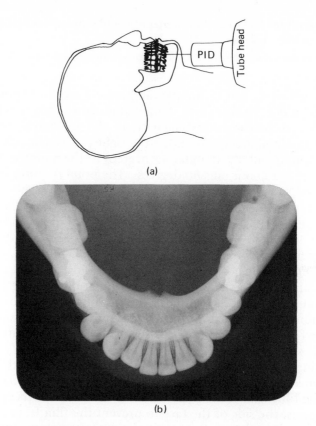

(a)

(b)

Fig. 14–4 (a) Diagram showing relationship of tube head and PID to occlusal film and patient for a cross-sectional view of the entire mandibular arch. Exposure side of the film faces mandibular arch with the widest dimension (longest) at right angles to the midsagittal plane. The central beam is directed perpendicularly to the occlusal plane through the inferior aspect of the mandible toward the center of the film. Slight modifications of this position must be made when the center of interest is in the canine or molar area or when a topographical view of the incisor area is desired. (b) Typical radiograph of cross-sectional view of the entire mandibular arch.

alternate method is to slide the film slightly to either side to obtain an oblique view of the teeth.

4.   Instruct the patient to close gently but firmly with his teeth against the film to immobilize it.

5.   Establish the horizontal angulation so that the central ray is parallel with the patient's midsagittal plane. Set the vertical angulation at minus 20 degrees to a line parallel to the plane of the floor. Thus, the total angle of the central ray in its relation to the film is approximately 65 degrees (45 degrees plus 20 degrees) because the patient is tilted back at a 45-degree angle.

6.   Direct the PID toward the center of the film through the point of entry at the point of the chin.

7.   Set the timer, adjust the controls as warranted, and make the exposure.

The Modified Mandibular Arch (Fig. 14–4)

Follow the same procedure as for the mandibular incisor survey, with these exceptions. A cross-sectional view is produced.

1.   Place the patient in a prone position and insert the film in the mouth with the longest dimension at right angles with the midsagittal plane.

2.   Establish the horizontal angulation at 0 degrees to the midsagittal plane and set the vertical angulation at 0 degrees and parallel to the plane of the floor.

3.   Direct the PID toward the center of the film through the point of entry, approximately 1 inch below the point of the chin.

4.   Set the timer, adjust the controls as warranted, and make the exposure.

The technique for the mandibular incisor survey, with slight changes in film placement and in horizontal and vertical angulations, will give a canine, molar, or floor of the mouth survey. To make the canine survey, first shift the film to the right or left side. Place the patient in a prone position and establish the horizontal angulation at about 45 degrees to the midsagittal plane, and the vertical angulation at 0 degrees to the plane of the floor. Then ask the patient to tilt his head slightly toward the side the film is on, and direct the central ray to the center of the film through the point of entry located directly under the canine along the inferior border of the mandible. To make the molar survey, use the same placement and angulation but alter the direction of the central ray so that the point of entry is directly under the mandibular first molar along the inferior border of the mandible. For a mouth floor survey, change the vertical angulation to minus 10 degrees. Direct the central ray at the center of the film through a point of entry approximately 1 inch below the point of the chin. A variation of this position can be used to locate calcified stones at the proximal end of Wharton's duct when they are hidden by the mylohyoid ridge. Turn the patient's head opposite to the side where the stone is suspected to be. This rotates the film to an angle of 90 degrees to the plane of the floor. Keep the same horizontal angulation but change the vertical angulation to minus 20 degrees, thus directing the central ray between the submaxillary gland and the lingual surface of the mandible.

If the patient is edentulous, position the film with its longest dimension at right angles with the midsagittal plane. The patient places his forefingers against the anterior border of the film to keep it from sliding forward and upward. If the patient has an upper denture, it may be left in the mouth to bite against the film.

Exposure procedures vary slightly according to the lesion or structure to be examined. For special results or in special situations, other head positions, film positions, or angulations may be used. Always use the fastest film; "D" speed is recommended. The patient's size, age, and the density of the bone structures must be considered when determining the exposure factors. Small intraoral cassettes with intensifying screens to reduce the exposure time may be used in special situations where dense cranial structures must be penetrated. For additional information on the more complex techniques see *Dental Roentgenology* by Ennis, Berry, and Phillips; *Dental Radiology* by Wuehrmann and Manson-Hing; and the booklet *X-Rays in Dentistry*.

bibliography

Ennis, Leroy M., Berry, Harrison M., and Phillips, James E. *Dental Roentgenology*, 6th ed. Philadelphia: Lea & Febiger, 1967.

O'Brien, Richard C. *Dental Radiography*, 2d ed. Philadelphia: W. B. Saunders Co., 1972.

Wainwright, William Ward. *Dental Radiology*, New York: McGraw-Hill Book Co., 1965.

Wuehrmann, Arthur H., and Manson-Hing, Lincoln R. *Dental Radiology*, 2d ed. St. Louis: The C. V. Mosby Co., 1969.

X-Rays in Dentistry, Rochester, N.Y.: Eastman Kodak Co., 1972.

15

radiography for children

importance of radiography for children

Children have the same basic needs for dental treatment as adults
have. It may sometimes be more difficult to treat young children
than adults, but the proper care of children's teeth is one of the dentist's basic responsibilities. From a materialistic point of view, too,
child patients are important to a growing practice. Treated as children, they may return as adults.

Unfortunately, many parents have not received adequate dental
education. Often they consider their childrens' teeth—particularly
the deciduous teeth—to be of little value. More and more parents,
however, are bringing in their children for regular dental inspections
and care, instead of only for emergencies. Dental education of the
parents is the key to solving problems caused by dental neglect of
children. Just as parents have been taught to accept vaccinations to
prevent disease, they must be taught to accept dental radiography to
reduce dental infections, dental caries, and disfigurations produced
by premature loss or prolonged retention of the teeth.

The dentist must direct his principal effort toward prevention rather
than correction of conditions caused by neglect. In the area of protection, radiography plays an important role, and perhaps no place in
dental practice is good radiography more important than with children. The best time to prevent dental problems is in childhood.

One frequent problem is infected teeth, which can seriously affect
a child's health. Hidden infections are often unsuspected. The longer
the source of infection remains undisclosed, the greater the effect on

the patient is likely to be. Deciduous teeth that are lost too early or retained too long may cause severe damage to the occlusion and other conditions that are difficult to correct later. Hidden lesions can only be detected by frequent periodic examinations including radiographs. Without them, proper diagnosis, intelligent treatment planning, and corrective measures are nearly impossible.

role of radiography in protecting the deciduous teeth

Many explanations are given for dental decay: bacterial action, faulty metabolism, excess acidity, neglect, faulty dental hygiene and heredity are some of them. Whatever the reason, one fact is clear— dental caries are most prevalent in children. Although the teeth form and begin to calcify in the prenatal stage, much of the rapid growth of teeth and facial bones takes place between birth and age six. It is during the formative years that the danger of permanent damage from dental neglect is greatest. At this stage, radiography is vital to both prevention and treatment. Through the periodic use of radiographs, the dentist can locate lesions in their beginning stages, check how well repairs are holding up, and see signs of further decay. Aside from dental caries, often unnoticed during a visual inspection, a radiograph shows the roots of the deciduous teeth as well as the developing permanent teeth within the alveolar bone. Timely and adequate dental treatment can often avert the premature loss of the deciduous teeth and the subsequent malocclusion, which can turn the child into a dental cripple. Probably over half of all tooth decay is overlooked without dental radiographs. Moreover disturbances in normal development, such as enamel hypoplasia (failure of the enamel to develop fully), anodontia (absence of teeth), the presence of dentigerous cysts (sacs or capsules containing fluid or producing teeth), supernumerary teeth, and a host of other conditions can be discovered only through radiographs.

when to expose radiographs on children

Unless an accident, toothache, or some other unusual circumstance causes a parent to bring his child to the dentist sooner, the first routine radiographic survey is usually made soon after all the deciduous teeth have erupted at age three. Ideally, children would receive routine dental inspections including radiographs even earlier, but today not enough dentists have the training in pedodontic procedures, the special equipment, or the psychological ability to work with very young children.

Several factors determine how often the child's teeth should be x-rayed and the size and number of films used. These include the cooperation and emotional stability of the child, the size of the mouth opening, the size and shape of the teeth and the dental arches, the operator's ability to position the film, the child's ability to retain the film and keep it still, and what information the dentist needs.

The second complete radiographic survey is usually made when the child is about six, the age when the first deciduous teeth fall out and the first of the permanent teeth erupt. The third survey is usually made at age nine, when the child has a combination of deciduous and permanent teeth. The fourth survey is generally made between the ages of twelve and fourteen, when the last deciduous teeth are lost. After this, film placement, size, and number are the same as for adults.

Except in emergencies, interproximal surveys are made at definite intervals between complete surveys to detect caries or other incipient lesions.

suggested techniques for pedodontic radiography

Methods for exposing radiographs on children are basically the same as those for adults. Though either the bisecting or paralleling technique can be employed, many children are too small for periapical film positioning or often cannot manage film holders.

Special consideration must be given to the child whose oral tissues are still in the formative stage. The oral mucosa of the young child is extremely sensitive to even the slightest pressure, especially when teeth are erupting or about to fall out. The newer soft film packets are helpful. If film holders are used they should not be too bulky or heavy. The plastic backing plate on some holders can be cut down to a smaller size. The oral cavity should be examined thoroughly for loose or erupting teeth, any parulis (fistula or gum boil), pulp polyps, herpes labialis (cold sores), aphthous ulcers (canker sores), or swollen salivary glands.

Small mouths and difficult behavior can make it hard to radiograph children. Competence helps, but the operator may also need to approach a child differently than he would an adult. Of course, children differ, just as adults do, in the size, shape, and location of anatomic structures, and in temperament and behavior as well. As always, technique and approach must fit the individual.

First impressions are always important and lasting. Unless an emergency makes it impossible, the young child's first visit to the dental office and the x-ray room should be pleasant and informative. Most children are extremely curious. Unless they have been frightened by an unpleasant experience in a hospital or medical or dental office, they are much more curious than apprehensive. Usually it is best to greet the child in the reception room and take him to the x-ray room without his parents. Talking to him and showing him some of the equipment to be used and radiographs of other children, will help in gaining his confidence. Since the child's first experience with radiography is such an important one, the visit should not be hurried and the operator must refrain from showing signs of impatience. The radiographic survey should be explained to the child in terms he can understand. For example, the x-ray machine can be explained as a camera that takes pictures of the teeth. The child should be given a film packet to feel and to handle. It may be unwrapped for him so that he can see where the film is. If a film holder is to be used, the child should be allowed to examine and handle it, perhaps to put it in his mouth to convince himself that it is not an object to be feared. The entire procedure should be carefully explained and rehearsed. If necessary, the operator should demonstrate on himself how to hold and keep it still. No exposure should be attempted before the child is emotionally prepared for the experience and understands what is to be done.

The easiest and most comfortable exposures—normally radiographs of the anterior teeth—should be exposed first to gain the child's confidence and get him used to having a film in his mouth. A young child's span of attention is not very long, and one must repeat instructions with each exposure. Young children are often fidgety and restless, so when the child is finally ready, exposures should be made as rapidly as possible.

Most children react favorably to the authority of a confident, capable operator. Occasionally, a stubborn or frightened child proves difficult to manage. If such a child does not respond to firmness, a parent or older brother or sister may accompany him into the x-ray room. In fact, if the child is too small to understand instructions or unable to hold the film, the parent may have to hold the film for him.

Only in emergencies should a child ever be forced to have any dental treatment. It is much better to delay until the second or third visit than to instill a lasting fear of dentistry. If the child remains uncooperative after the third visit, a telephone call to his physician may be advisable to arrange for sedation. The sedative should be administered shortly before the appointment.

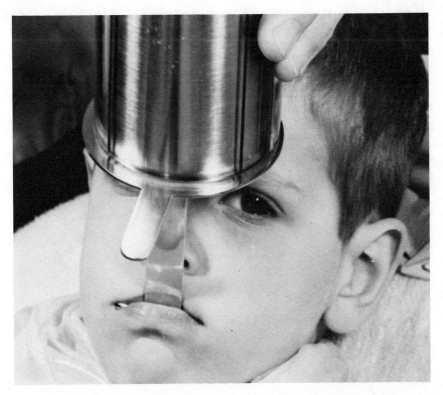

Fig. 15–1 Child with a "Precision" (Elcan) anterior child instrument in place.
Steel cone liner is used to reduce cone scatter radiation and rectangular window
in steel shield acts as a further collimating device. (Courtesy of Precision X-Ray
Company.)

Both intraoral and extraoral films are used in making the radiographic survey on a young child. The choice of film size and type
depends upon the age of the patient and the area to be examined. As
a rule, best results are obtained on a young patient when a combination of techniques and films is used. Periapical film placement is not
always possible and extraoral films provide much essential information
about the growth and development of the jaws.

One problem in using periapical films is the distortion caused by
the flatness of the palate and floor of the mouth in children. Because
of it, films lie flatter than they do in the mouths of most adults. This
position results in an increase in the size of the angle between the
teeth and the films, requiring an adjustment to compensate. When
bisecting methods are used, the steepness of the vertical angulation
is increased.

This problem can be solved by use of paralleling methods. Child-
size holders can be used (Fig. 15–1), or the biteblocks on the X-C-P

instruments can be modified by reducing the size of the backing plate with shears or a knife to accommodate the #0 or #00 film. If the child objects to the film holder in his mouth or has difficulty biting hard enough to stabilize it, have the child hold the film with his thumb or index finger, guided by the radiographer. When the child is too small to be seated in the dental chair, his mother can sit in the chair with the child on her lap and hold the film for him. Under no circumstances should the radiographer hold the film packet.

Because the child is smaller, his gonads are much closer to the source of radiation than are those of adults. A lead apron should always be placed over him. Special small lead aprons are available. As the bone structure on a child is smaller and less dense than that of an adult, average exposure time can be reduced by about one-third to one-half.

film requirements for the pedodontic radiographic survey

Various combinations of periapical, interproximal occlusal, or extraoral films are suggested, depending on the child. As usual, the survey should be thorough but as comfortable as possible. Ideally, the survey includes a minimum of twelve radiographs, ten periapical, and two interproximal exposures. The periapical films are exposed in each of the four molar and canine areas, and in the maxillary and mandibular incisor areas. One interproximal film is exposed in the molar areas of each side. Occlusal and extraoral exposures are included when requested by the dentist. However, small size, tongue resistance, and gagging can be a problem in small children and occlusal and extraoral films make an acceptable substitute on a three- or four-year-old child (Fig. 15-2). At this age, it is often inadvisable to expose more than four films, one occlusal film in each jaw in the area of the anterior teeth, and an extraoral film of each of the lateral jaw areas. Although not as good as periapical or interproximal films in detecting caries, these show the formation of the permanent tooth buds and the relationship between deciduous and developing permanent dentition. Most children at that age do not object to occlusal and extraoral films, as they cause a minimum of discomfort.

During the second radiographic survey at age six, the first permanent teeth have begun to erupt. Since the child is now more mature, it may be possible to make the periapical exposure of all tooth areas, particularly if he had interproximal radiographs made during periodic inspections at age four and five. If using periapical films is still not

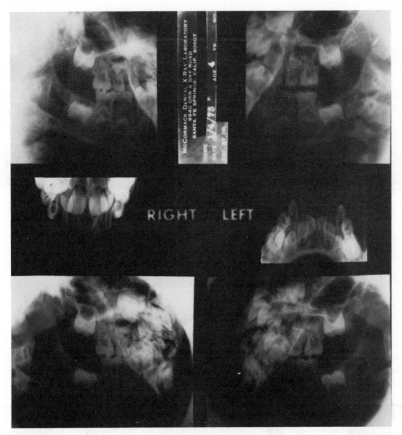

Fig. 15-2 Combination of occlusal radiograph of incisal area and extraoral lateral jaw radiographs of the posterior areas of a four-year-old child. (Courtesy of Mc-Cormack Dental X-Ray Laboratory.)

feasible, the survey can be made with a minimum of six films; two occlusally, two extraorally, and two interproximally (Fig. 15-3).

At nine, the child has a mixed dentition. This examination may be made with as few as six and as many as twenty or more exposures. The larger #2 periapical films can often be used at this age; however, the smaller film sizes are most frequently used (Fig. 15-4).

Between twelve and fourteen years of age, the child gets all his permanent teeth except the third molars. It is during this preadolescent period that growth is most rapid and metabolic changes occur that heighten the possibility of dental caries and increase the need for vigilance and preventive care. This fourth survey should be made with a minimum of fourteen periapical and two interproximal films. It is the same as that for the adult and larger films can be used.

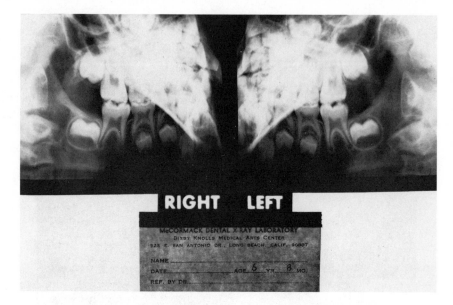

Fig. 15-3 Right and left lateral jaw-type radiographs of six-year-old child. When accompanied with an occlusal view of the maxillary and mandibular incisal areas, and the right and left interproximal (bitewing) radiographs, the normal minimal diagnostic requirements can be met. (Courtesy of McCormack Dental X-Ray Laboratory.)

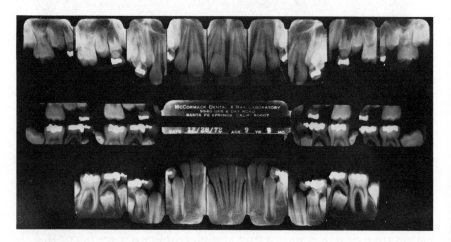

Fig. 15-4 Complete radiographic periapical and interproximal series on a nine-year-old child. Depending on the size of the child, fewer films or films of several sizes may be used to make such a survey. (Courtesy of McCormack Dental X-Ray Laboratory.)

interproximal and periapical exposures for children

With few minor exceptions to compensate for the child's smaller mouth, the same technical procedures described in Chapters 12 and 13 are used when exposing radiographs on children. The main difference is in the use of smaller films and shorter exposure times. In addition, in some areas a slightly steeper vertical angulation than is customary in adults is used to compensate for the shorter teeth and the flatter palate and more shallow floor of the mouth during bisecting. Other minor changes in technique are listed below for each of the exposures commonly made in a full-mouth series of radiographs for children.

The Posterior Interproximal Survey (Fig. 15-5)

Only one interproximal film is required on each side unless the second permanent molars have already erupted. If possible, the front edge of the film should cover the distal portion of the mandibular canine. Corners of the film packet are softened so as not to bruise the delicate oral tissues. If the bisecting technique is used, the vertical angulation is increased from plus 8 to plus 10 degrees—to compensate for the greater bending of the upper half of the film packet to conform to the reduced curvature of the child's palate. Depending on the age and the size of the child, the exposure time is normally one-third less than used for making interproximal or periapical exposures on an adult. If the child is very small, the milliamperage and kilovoltage may also be reduced.

The Mandibular Incisor Survey (Fig. 15-6)

Depending on the technique, the film is placed in the mouth with its longest dimension vertically and held in place by the child's finger, or it is placed vertically in the biteblock on which the child closes. The average vertical angulation for bisecting is minus 20 to 25 degrees. Center the film at the midline and allow about 1/8 inch of the film to protrude above the incisal edge to leave an incisal margin. Refer back to Chapter 12 for procedures of the periapical exposures.

The Mandibular Canine Survey (Fig. 15-7)

Except for minor positioning and angulation changes, follow the same procedures as for the mandibular incisors. The front edge of the film

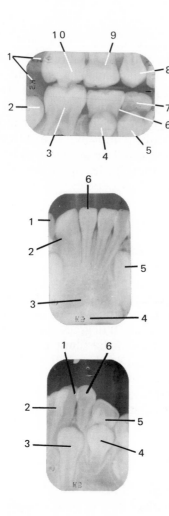

Fig. 15-5 Posterior interproximal radiograph of mixed dentition: 1. Alveolar bone; 2. unerupted mandibular permanent second molar; 3. permanent mandibular first molar — fully erupted; 4. erupting mandibular second premolar; 5. erupting mandibular first premolar; 6. mandibular second deciduous molar — roots almost resorbed; 7. mandibular first deciduous molar — roots totally resorbed and ready to exfoliate; 8. newly erupted maxillary permanent first premolar; 9. deciduous maxillary second molar; 10. fully-erupted maxillary permanent first molar.

Fig. 15-6 Mandibular incisor area exposed on small #0 film: 1. Deciduous canine (cuspid); 2. permanent lateral incisor (permanent) — tooth appears wider than it actually is through distortion of film caused by placement in narrow arch; 3. genial tubercles — radiopaque circular area within alveolar bone; 4. inferior border of mandible — radiopaque band at bottom of film; 5. unerupted permanent canine; 6. fully-erupted permanent central incisor.

Fig. 15-7 Radiograph of mandibular canine (cuspid) area exposed on small #0 film: 1. Permanent lateral incisor; 2. permanent central incisor — radiopaque area between teeth is caused by overlapping of the teeth; 3. permanent canine in process of erupting; 4. permanent first premolar — root has just started to form but crown is already pushing against roots of deciduous first molar; 5. deciduous first molar — roots are almost resorbed; 6. deciduous canine — root is just beginning to be resorbed.

should extend forward to cover the distal portion of the mandibular lateral incisor. Increase the average vertical angulation to minus 25 to minus 30 degrees if using the bisecting method.

The Mandibular Molar Survey (Fig. 15-8)

The film is held with its longest dimension horizontally by the child's finger or is placed horizontally in the biteblock on which the child closes. The film is centered over the mandibular molars. If possible

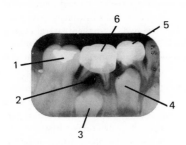

Fig. 15-8 Radiograph of mandibular molar area exposed on #0 film: 1. Fully-erupted permanent molar with occlusal metal (amalgam) restoration; 2. radiolucent area under deciduous tooth indicates bone loss due to infection; 3. crown of permanent second premolar; 4. erupting permanent first premolar — root only starting to form; 5. deciduous first molar with steel crown (light radiopacity because crown is very thin) showing radiopaque area under crown indicating some form of cement used in vital pulpotomy — mesial root still present but distal root is completely resorbed; 6. deciduous second molar with steel crown and evidence of vital pulpotomy (radiopaque) and infection under tooth (radiolucent).

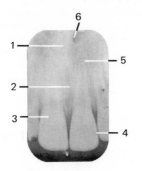

Fig. 15-9 Radiograph of maxillary incisor area exposed on #0 film: 1. Nasal septum — radiopaque bone area; 2. incisive foramen — round slightly-radiolucent area; 3. fully-erupted permanent right central incisor; 4. incipient cavity on distal of left permanent central incisor (radiolucent); 5. apex of root not fully formed; 6. nasal fossa — radiolucent area at top of film.

the front edge of the film should cover the distal portion of the mandibular canine. Increase the average vertical angulation to between minus 15 to minus 20 degrees.

The Maxillary Incisor Survey (Fig. 15-9)

Follow similar procedures as for the mandibular incisor survey. The film is positioned with its longest dimension vertically and centered at the midline. Increase the average vertical angulation to about plus 45 to plus 50 degrees if using the bisecting method.

The Maxillary Canine Survey (Fig. 15-10)

Follow the same procedure as for the maxillary incisor survey, but shift the film laterally so that it is centered over the long axis of the maxillary canine. Place the front edge of the film so that it covers

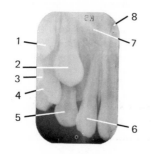

Fig. 15–10   Radiograph of maxillary canine (cuspid) area exposed on #0 film: 1. Erupting permanent second premolar; 2. unerupted permanent canine; 3. mesial edge of crown of second deciduous molar; 4. erupted first permanent premolar crown; 5. deciduous canine — root partially resorbed permanent canine underneath lacks sufficient space for normal eruption; 6. permanent lateral incisor; 7. floor of nasal fossa — narrow radiopaque band; 8. nasal fossa — darker radiolucent area.

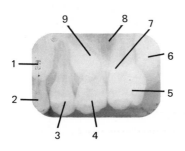

Fig. 15–11   Radiograph of maxillary molar area exposed with #0 film: 1. Erupting permanent canine; 2. deciduous canine — root partially resorbed; 3. fully-erupted first premolar; 4. deciduous second molar — tooth being bypassed and root still intact; 5. fully erupted permanent first molar; 6. unerupted crown of permanent second molar still covered with bone; 7. white radiopaque line is inferior border of maxillary sinus; 8. maxillary sinus — radiopaque area; 9. permanent second premolar not following path of normal eruption — tooth directed buccally and distally.

the distal half of the maxillary lateral incisor. For the bisecting technique the average vertical angulation ranges from plus 55 to plus 60 degrees.

   The Maxillary Molar Survey (Fig. 15–11)

As with the mandibular molar exposure, position the film horizontally over the molar area with the front edge covering the distal border of the maxillary canine. For the bisecting technique, the average vertical angulation ranges from plus 30 to plus 55 degrees.

   When making any of these exposures for the first time, review how to use the film holders (Chapter 12) and modify these procedures for use with the child patient. In most cases, either the bisecting or paralleling technique can be used successfully.

the occlusal survey for children

   The occlusal technique is the same for children as for adults, except that the exposure time is decreased. Although the film may be positioned several ways, the maxillary and mandibular incisor surveys described in Chapter 14 are the two variations used most often if the large occlusal film is used. When the child's mouth is too small to accommodate the occlusal film, a smaller film is positioned in whatever direction that will give the maximum coverage of the desired area.

the lateral jaw survey for children

The technique for making the lateral jaw exposure is fully described in Chapter 17. The exposure can be made with any size extraoral film or with an occlusal film placed against the cheek when the child is small or the dentist is interested only in a limited area of the teeth. If an occlusal film is used, line up the longest dimension of the film so that it is flush with the lower border of the mandible and line up the front edge of the film with the corner of the mouth. Place the tube side of the film against the cheek and ask the child to hold it with his fingers or palm of the hand. Use the ala-tragus line as a guide to parallel the child's occlusal plane with the plane of the floor, and press against the top of his head gently until the head is tipped about 20 degrees toward the side of the film. Then ask the child to close his mouth so that the upper and lower teeth touch each other and direct the central ray through a point of entry toward the center of the film at a vertical angulation of about minus 10 degrees from a point slightly behind and below the angle of the opposite mandible.

When extraoral films are used, the size depends on the size of the child's head and the structures that the dentist wishes to include. A cardboard exposure holder loaded with non-screen film or a cassette with screen film may be used. If the child is small, the light-weight cardboard exposure holder may be easiest for him to hold. However, the exposure time can be shortened when the heavier cassette with intensifying screens is used. In either case, place the tube side toward the cheek and center the film so that it covers all structures of interest. Several head positions are used with extraoral films; the child may be upright or prone, or the cassette may be laid flat on a table and the child sits in front of it and bends his head until his face contacts the tube side. With some practice each operator develops his favorite technique.

bibliography

Ennis, Leroy M., Berry, Harrison M., and Phillips, James E.. *Dental Roentgenology*, 6th ed. Philadelphia: Lea & Febiger, 1969.

O'Brien, Richard C. *Dental Radiography*, 2d ed. Philadelphia: W. B. Saunders Co., 1972.

Peterson, Shailer. *Clinical Dental Hygiene*, 3d ed. St. Louis: The
C. V. Mosby Co., 1968.

Updegrave, William J. *New Horizons in Periapical and Interproximal Radiography*, Elgin, Ill.: Rinn Corporation, 1971.

Wainwright, William Ward. *Dental Radiology*, New York: McGraw-Hill Book Co., 1965.

Wilkins, Esther M. *Clinical Practice of the Dental Hygienist*, 3d ed.
Philadelphia: Lea & Febiger, 1969.

X-Rays in Dentistry, Rochester, N.Y.: Eastman Kodak Co., 1972.

16
radiography
for the edentulous patient

the importance of radiography for the edentulous

A complete examination of the edentulous patient includes radiographs along with the visual and digital inspection. Preventive radiography often is of great benefit to the fully and partially edentulous because the normal appearance of the arches (dental ridges) may conceal problems underneath. Most edentulous persons have lost their teeth through neglect of decay, infection, or untreated periodontal conditions. Though the teeth have been extracted and the ridges have healed in a satisfactory manner, infection may not have been totally eradicated. It can usually be detected and eliminated only if radiographs are made before prosthetic treatments begin. Occasionally, too, oral malignancies existing in elderly patients are first detected on radiographs. Unfortunately, many edentulous patients do not understand why radiographs are needed. Sometimes even the dentist is positive that since the patient has been wearing dentures for years, everything must be in order.

Potential sources of difficulty may be present in a substantial number of edentulous ridges that interfere with the comfortable wearing of prosthetic appliances. A survey of over a thousand edentulous patients conducted at the University of Pennsylvania Dental Clinic[1] showed that this group of patients had a total of 355 roots imbedded within the ridges, 21 of which were associated with radiolucent areas.

---

1. L. M. Ennis and H. M. Berry, *"The Necessity for Routine Examinations in the Edentulous Mouth," Journal of Oral Surgery,* **7** (1948), 3–19.

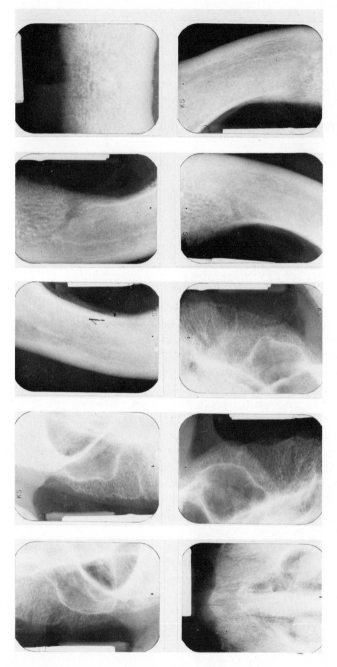

Fig. 16-1 Edentulous survey made with ten standard #2 periapical films. All exposures were made with the paralleling technique as evidenced by the radiopaque outline cast by the biteblocks. (Courtesy of UCLA School of Dentistry.)

Fourteen of these patients had residual areas of infection, 32 had impacted or unerupted teeth, 5 had supernumerary teeth, 10 had cysts, and 12 had foreign bodies imbedded in the ridge. These included bits of amalgam, buckshot from a hunting accident, tips of broken root canal broaches, and remnants of impression paste forced into the antrum (sinus) when immediate impressions were taken. Nine had stones in Wharton's duct, 5 had odontomas (tumors derived from tissues involved in tooth formation), 13 had sequestra (pieces of dead bone separated from sound bone in necrosis) at the crest of the ridge, one had an unsuspected fracture of the alveolar process. The radiographs of the three patients revealed suspicious areas on which biopsies were made, and the presence of a carcinoma (malignant tumor of connective tissue origin) was confirmed in 2 of these patients.

These are only some of the conditions that may exist under an apparently healthy ridge. The list is imposing enough to suggest that making a radiographic survey on an edentulous patient should be considered routine.

film requirements for the edentulous survey

Several methods involving various combinations of intraoral, occlusal, or extraoral films are commonly used for a radiographic survey of the edentulous mouth. Some dentists prefer to use 14 periapical films—7 for the maxillary and 7 for the mandibular ridges—placing the films over the same areas of the ridges as they would if the teeth were still present; others use only 10 films (Fig. 16-1). Still others prefer a total of seven films: two occlusal films (one in each arch), and five periapical films (one in each of the four posterior regions and one in the mandibular incisor region).

In addition to being faster to make and subjecting the patient to less radiation, the latter method has the advantage of pinpointing the location of root fragments, lesions, or other objects because two planes of reference are available instead of one. The occlusal film shows a larger section of the jaw structures in relationship to each other and the buccolingual location of teeth or lesions in a horizontal plane whereas the periapical films show them in a vertical plane.

The occlusal radiograph serves as an excellent guide in establishing the relative position of various structures or lesions to recognizable landmarks; however, it may not show some details that periapical radiographs do. Periapical films are used in all four molar areas to supplement the occlusal film, because anatomical restrictions often keep the film from being inserted far enough back to include the third molar area. It is in this region that broken root fragments or unerupted teeth are most likely to be discovered. The anterior region of the mandible is also radiographed, because the small size of the mandibular incisors and the denseness of the bone near the front of the mandible often make the identification of small root fragments very difficult on occlusal exposures.

Additional films may be used to supplement such a seven-film survey if the presence of some unsuspected object is detected and more information is required. Two other effective methods for viewing large edentulous areas involve the use of extraoral films. The conventional x-ray machine may be used to make a lateral jaw exposure on each side, or, in offices that have a panoramic x-ray unit, the survey can be made on a single film (Fig. 16–2). As is the case with occlusal film, these extraoral films can be supplemented with other films if abnormal or unusual conditions are discovered.

techniques for making the edentulous survey

Fundamentally, the technique for exposing the 14 edentulous regions of the mandible or maxillae are very similar to the suggested procedures for exposing the periapical regions that were described in Chapter 12. These exposures can be made with any size periapical film, but the standard #2 film is generally the film of choice. Either the bisecting or the paralleling technique may be employed. Whichever technique is used, the important thing is to get clear images of

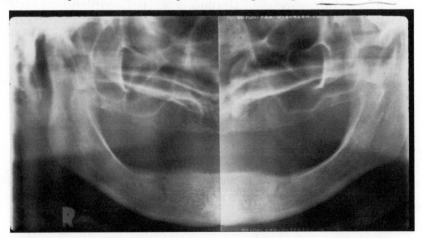

Fig. 16-2 Complete edentulous survey made on panoramic type x-ray machine. Relationship of the maxillary and mandibular structures are shown on a single film. (Courtesy of UCLA School of Dentistry.)

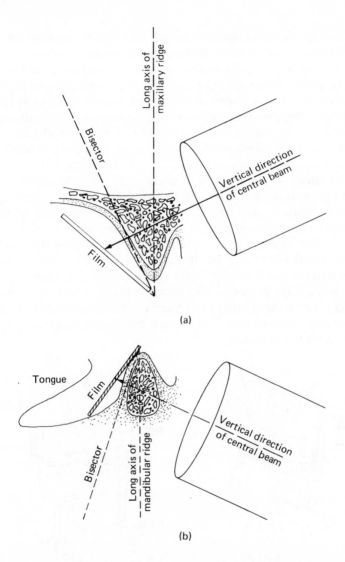

(a)

(b)

Fig. 16-3 Diagrams showing the relationship of the film to the ridge of an edentulous patient. The film packet lies much flatter in the mouth when teeth are
missing. Films are placed vertically for anterior and horizontally for posterior
exposures. Unless film holders are used, the film is stabilized by the patient's
thumb or index finger. When the rules of bisecting are followed, an imaginary
line can be drawn vertically through the ridge to substitute for the long axis of the
teeth formerly in the ridge. As in bisecting, the central beam is directed perpendicularly to the bisector to determine the correct vertical angulation. The correct
horizontal angulation is difficult to determine in the edentulous patient; however,
it is not a major consideration since the absence of teeth eliminates overlapping.
(a) Maxillary edentulous ridge; (b) mandibular edentulous ridge.

all fully or partially edentulous regions. The size of the film, or the number of films used, is of secondary importance.

Several minor modifications in technique are required for x-raying edentulous areas. Normally, the teeth serve as landmarks to guide film placement. Also, the center of interest is no longer the teeth, but the ridge. Because the teeth are no longer present, visualizing the bisecting plane and establishing horizontal and vertical planes are more difficult, particularly when the bisecting technique is used. Fortunately, a fair amount of leeway in horizontal angulation is permissible, because the absence of teeth eliminates the problem of overlapping tooth images. In the bisecting method, since the long axes of the teeth can no longer be used as a guide, one determines vertical angulation by bisecting the angle formed between the record-ing plane of the film and an imaginary line through the ridge that substitutes for the long axes of the teeth (Fig. 16–3). Unfortunately, when the patient holds the film with his fingers, it lies much flatter than when teeth are present. This often results in a failure to show all the details of a small area, and in some, dimensional distortion of the visible structure occurs. However, acceptable radiographs can be produced with the bisecting method.

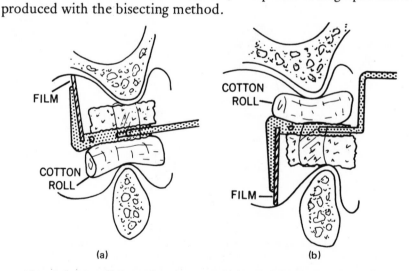

(a)   (b)

Fig. 16–4 When all the teeth are missing, cotton rolls, blocks of styrofoam or a combination of both can be used with the X-C-P instruments. Their thickness will determine the amount of film coverage of the edentulous ridges. The instrument is positioned in the mouth with the film parallel to the ridge area being examined. The patient closes stabilizing and holding the film in position and the standard procedures are followed. (a) Maxillary posterior region. The film holder is rotated so the film is directed down for the mandibular areas. (b) Mandibular anterior region. The film holder is rotated so that the film is directed upward for the maxillary posterior areas. (Courtesy of Rinn Corporation, Dental X-Ray Division.)

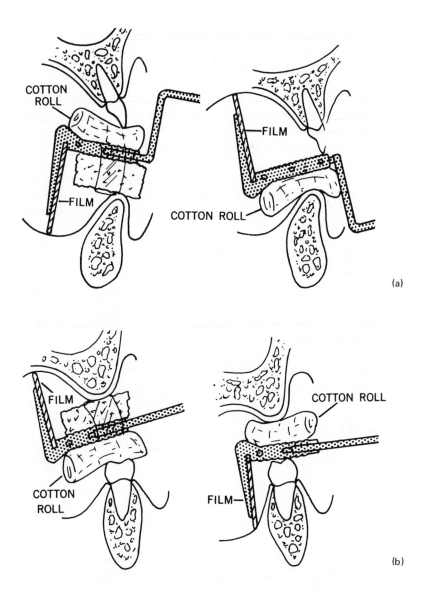

Fig. 16-5 The versatile X-C-P instruments can also be used in radiography of the partially edentulous mouths by substituting a cotton roll or block of styrofoam (or a similar radiolucent material) for the space normally occupied by the crowns of the missing teeth and then following standard procedures. (a) Edentulous mandibular anterior region. Opposite placement for the maxillary region. (b) Edentulous maxillary posterior region. Rotate instrument opposite way for the mandibular posterior areas. (Courtesy of Rinn Corporation, Dental X-Ray Division.)

The paralleling technique usually gives better results. Radiographic detail is improved and dimensional distortion is minimized when film holders, properly supported by cotton rolls or styrofoam blocks, are used to hold the film parallel to the long axis of the ridge.

When all the teeth are missing, cotton rolls, blocks of styrofoam, or a combination can be used with ordinary biteblocks or film holders as the X-C-P instruments. The thickness of the cotton rolls or styrofoam will determine the coverage of the edentulous ridge. The film is placed vertically in the anterior biteblocks and horizontally in the posterior biteblocks. Since definite landmarks are seldom present, one must guess the best film position. Obviously, the incisor and molar regions are easiest to locate. Shifting the film distally or mesially is necessary to locate the canine and premolar regions. The biteblock or film holder is then placed in the mouth with the film parallel to the ridge being examined. The patient closes, holding the film in position. The final step is to direct the rays horizontally and vertically toward the center of the film perpendicularly to the mean tangent of the facial side of the ridge and to the plane of the film (Fig. 16-4). As a rule, 25 percent less exposure is required for an edentulous area than for one with teeth.

One can also modify this technique for use with the partially edentulous patient by substituting cotton rolls or a block of styrofoam for the space normally occupied by the crowns of the missing teeth and then following the standard procedures (Fig. 16-5).

The dentist may prefer to use larger films to make the edentulous survey. The procedure for making this survey was described in Chapter 14. The methods for exposing the lateral jaw and the panoramic films is described in Chapter 17.

bibliography

Ennis, Leroy M., Berry, Harrison M., and Phillips, James E. *Dental Roentgenology,* 6th ed. Philadelphia: Lea & Febiger, 1967.

O'Brien, Richard C. *Dental Radiography,* 2d ed. Philadelphia: W. B. Saunders Co., 1972.

Updegrave, William J. *New Horizons in Periapical and Interproximal Radiography,* Elgin, Ill.: Rinn Corporation, 1971.

Wainwright, William Ward. *Dental Radiology,* New York: McGraw-Hill Book Co., 1965.

Wuehrmann, Arthur H., and Manson-Hing, Lincoln R. *Dental Radiology,* 2d ed. St. Louis: The C. V. Mosby Co., 1969.

17

extraoral radiography

types and uses of extraoral radiography

Extraoral films are used to show a larger area than an intraoral film can show, when swelling or injury makes intraoral film placement impossible, when a child will not tolerate films intraorally, and when one wants to show the entire dentition and adjacent structures on a single film. Extraoral radiographs may be used alone or with periapical, interproximal, or occlusal radiographs. Sometimes panoramic films or intraoral films (usually occlusal) are used to make extraoral exposures. The latter technique can be modified to make exposures of the third molar areas. Chapter 15 describes making extraoral exposures on children with occlusal film. The most common method of making extraoral radiographs is to use 5 in. by 7 in. or 8 in. by 10 in. extraoral films to show large portions of the mandible or the maxilla, a complete posteroanterior view of the skull, a facial profile, or the temporomandibular joint. Such radiographs are normally of more value to the oral surgeon, the orthodontist, or the prosthodontist than to the general practitioner. Special purpose techniques are described in advanced radiography texts and professional journals.

The posteroanterior and lateral jaw surveys provide an overall view of the facial bones and jaw structures. They are extremely helpful to the oral surgeon in determining the extent of fractures, bone diseases, malignancies, the presence of foreign bodies, and other items of interest.

The radiograph of the temporomandibular joint is essential in determining the extent of damage caused by tooth loss, injuries, or diseases of this region.

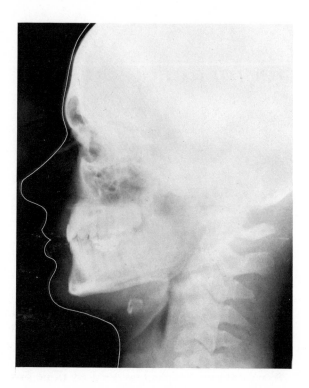

Fig. 17-1   Radiograph profile exposed in extraoral cassette. Radiograph was
underdeveloped to enhance the outlines of the soft tissues. Template can be
made by cutting along the image of the facial outline which then serves as a guide
in maintaining the profile.

The posteroanterior and lateral radiographs of the bones and tooth
structures and the profile radiographs of the soft structures show the
orthodontist the anatomy of the jaw, the growth and development
of the dentition, and provide a record of the changes produced by
orthodontic treatment.

The prosthodontist frequently makes two facial profile radiographs
before the teeth are extracted—one to record the profile of the patient
and the other to record the normal relationship of the teeth to each
other when the jaws are closed normally. To do this, he places two
films in an exposure holder and exposes them together but develops
them differently. A template to be held against the face as a guide
in maintaining the original contour and vertical dimensions of the
face can be made by cutting along the outline of the profile on one
of the radiographs. The other radiograph is kept as a record. Postoperative radiographs are also frequently used by the prosthodontists
to compare the original conditions with the results (Fig. 17-1).

As the larger extraoral films are packaged differently from intra-oral films, they require special handling in the darkroom. Types of films and techniques for loading them are fully explained in Chapter 7.

Many film positions and techniques require special equipment and a sound knowledge of the anatomic structures through which the radiation beam is directed. Such special equipment is especially required for radiographs on physically and emotionally handicapped patients. Most of these exposures are made in hospitals, x-ray laboratories, or oral surgery offices by highly experienced operators. Only a few of the easier-to-make exposures are described in this book. For further information about extraoral exposures, consult the Bibliography at the end of this chapter, as well as the books in the dental school library.

exposures with extraoral films

Many methods can be used to make radiographic surveys of the head and face. Depending on the equipment available, the patient may be upright in a standard dental chair, lying prone in a contour chair or on a special table, or bending over a table and placing his head on it for stability. In the latter case, plastic bags filled with sand may be used to prop the head at a desired angle and keep it stable during the exposure. It is not within the scope of this book to describe all these techniques. Because contour chairs and other special equipment are not used in many offices, the descriptions that follow assume the use of a standard dental chair.

The Lateral Jaw Survey

The lateral jaw survey is the most frequently made extraoral exposure. It is especially valuable to use with children (Fig. 17–2), with patients

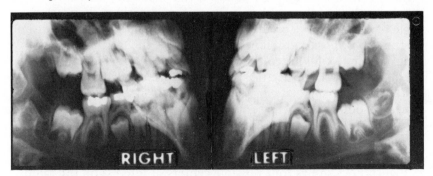

Fig. 17–2 Typical lateral jaw radiograph of a child with a mixed dentition. This exposure is generally made with 5″ × 7″ film on adults.

who have fractures or swelling, with patients who are too young or senile to hold intraoral films, and patients with other special problems. The lateral jaw exposure is often made to evaluate the condition of the bone or locate larger lesions or impacted teeth. Some practitioners consider the lateral jaw survey an essential adjunct to a full-mouth periapical series.

Because the amount of bone that must be penetrated by the x-radiation is relatively small in the lateral jaw regions, one may use the easier-to-hold cardboard exposure holder with non-screen film. Many routinely use cassettes with screen film. Either procedure is acceptable.

One satisfactory technique is to seat the patient upright in the dental chair with the midsagittal plane of his head perpendicular and the occlusal plane parallel to the floor. This can be done rapidly by using the ala-tragus line as a guide. Some radiographers prefer a slight tilt of the head (about 10 to 20 degrees) toward the side on which the film is held. Whether the film is positioned with its longest dimension parallel or perpendicular to the lower border of the body of the mandible depends on the size of the film used. Ideally, the front edge of the film should protrude slightly beyond the tip of the nose and the chin. Normally the region of the first molars will be near the center of the film. The patient presses the tube side of the exposure holder or cassette firmly against the cheek with the palm of his hand, and curves his fingers so that they rest on the top of his head.

Unfortunately, a true projection of the central ray is not possible in the lateral jaw survey. Some magnification and dimensional distortion are unavoidable, because true paralleling is impossible for anatomic reasons. Although the rays can be directed perpendicularly toward the film in a horizontal plane, this cannot be done in the vertical plane because overlapping of the right and left sides would occur. Thus, depending on whether the center of interest is in the region of the body or of the ramus of the mandible, the center of the PID is directed at the point of entry, either slightly underneath the angle of the mandible or an inch higher and slightly behind the ramus on the side opposite the film. In either case, the trajectory of the central beam is oblique to the vertical plane. A larger area of the maxilla and mandible can be surveyed by projecting the beam from underneath the angle of the mandible than from behind the ramus. However, doing this increases the dimensional distortion because the vertical angulation of the x-radiation is not as steep; therefore more detail of a limited area is observed when the point of entry is behind the ramus.

Figure 17-3 shows four possible centers of interest on the radiograph: the ramus area, the molars, the premolars, and the incisors.

To change the center of interest, one varies the angle at which the film is held against the face and the direction of the PID, so that the beam of radiation is directed perpendicularly to the desired area, usually at the level of the occlusal plane. The short PID is used; however, the target-film distance is at least 5 inches greater than when the film is placed intraorally because the source of the radiation is at the opposite side of the face. Before making the exposure, ask the patient to thrust his mandible forward so that the vertebrae will not be superimposed on mandibular structures. Estimate the target-film distance and the density of the structures to determine the exposure factors. Follow the manufacturer's recommendations on exposure time according to type of film used.

The Facial Profile Survey

To make a facial profile exposure, seat the patient in the same manner as for the lateral jaw exposure. Depending on whether only the bone tissues or the details of the soft tissues are to be examined, either one

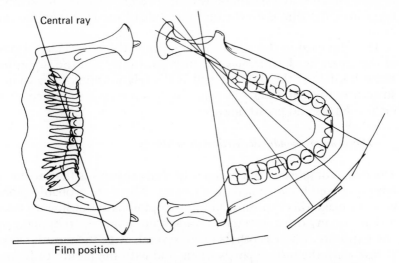

Fig. 17-3 X-ray beam direction for the lateral jaw projection. Rays strike the film obliquely in the vertical plane but should be perpendicular in the horizontal plane. A true lateral projection of an entire side of the jaw is not possible since the image of the opposite side would be superimposed on it. The lateral jaw projection must be made with some oblique angulation. The beam of radiation can be directed toward the area of interest from two basic directions underneath the mandible opposite the one being radiographed or behind the mandible opposite the one being radiographed. Modifications are possible by directing the beam from any area between these basic positions. (From Wuehrmann, Arthur H., and Manson-Hing, Lincoln R. *Dental Radiology*, 2d ed. St. Louis: The C. V. Mosby Co., 1969.)

or two films are loaded into an 8 in. by 10 in. exposure holder or cassette with par (average) speed intensifying screen. If the objective is to concentrate on the soft tissues, the film is developed for only 1¼ minutes at 68°F. Full development for about 4½ minutes at 68°F. is required to show the bone structures fully.

The patient holds the exposure holder or cassette with one hand against the middle and the other at the lower front border. Additional support is gained by resting the shortest dimension on the patient's shoulder. Center the film with the tube side over the zygomatic arch and make sure that the front edge protrudes about an inch past the tip of the nose.

Set the exposure time as directed by the manufacturer for the type of film used. Instruct the patient to keep his jaws in an at rest position. The average target-film distance for this exposure is 72 inches, which is about the maximum distance that the extension arm on most x-ray machines can be placed. Place the PID at 0-degrees angulation to direct the beam perpendicularly to the recording plane of the film. Raise or lower the dental chair so that both the center of the film and the PID are on the same level. As with all extraoral exposures, the film is on the opposite side of the face than the tube head.

The film used in this survey is large enough to give a lateral view of the entire head. It shows the anteroposterior and the superoinferior borders of the skull, as well as the relationship of anatomic structures to each other. That is why this survey is so valuable to orthodontists and prosthodontists.

The Temporomandibular Articulation Survey

The most complex of the frequently made surveys is that of the temporomandibular articulation (joint). There are probably more ways to make this exposure and more opinions about how to expose it than for any other extraoral radiograph. Some dentists make only one exposure, whereas others make several—with the mouth closed at rest, with the mouth partly open, and with the mouth fully open (Fig. 17–4). Because this exposure is made from the opposite side, the central beam has to pass first through a series of bones and soft structures. Therefore, the exposure requires extreme care and accuracy in adjusting the cassette to the head position and directing the PID so that the rays will strike the film at the best angle.

A simple technique is to have the patient upright in the dental chair. As the area to be examined is relatively small, a common practice is to use a single large film and make several exposures on it.

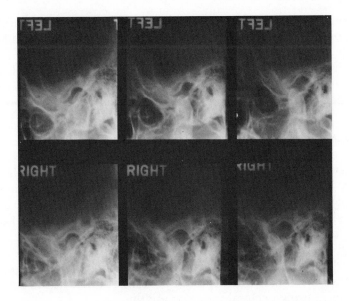

Fig. 17-4 Serial radiographs of the temporomandibular articulation showing the head of the condyle in the glenoid fossa with the mouth closed, in the at rest position, and with the mouth open. A stabilizing device of some type is generally required to hold the patient's head in a firm position while the cassette is moved for each exposure on the same side. Such equipment for serial radiography is not available in most offices; however, single exposures can readily be made using similar techniques as for the lateral jaw exposures. (Courtesy of McCormack Dental X-Ray Laboratory.)

Parts of the film are covered with lead so that only one part of the film is exposed each time. Thus three or four exposures, with the head of the condyle in a different position each time, can be made consecutively on the same film. Some dentists use an occlusal film when a single survey only is required. To make the exposure, use a short PID at a target-film distance of about 15 inches and direct the central ray at a vertical angulation of about plus 20 degrees to the center of the part of the film that is not covered with lead. Caution the patient not to move or change position and follow the manufacturer's suggestions for the exposure time.

The disadvantage of this technique is that it is difficult to stabilize the patient's head and prevent movement. Moreover, it is difficult to repeat the same exposure and get identical results. For this reason, many prefer to prop up and support the patient's head.

The temporomandibular survey provides radiographs of the temporomandibular joint (TMJ). Disturbances of this articulation are very common and cause much patient discomfort. A clear radiograph, or series of radiographs, showing the head of the mandibular condyle in the glenoid fossa of the temporal bone is essential for the dentist to make a diagnostic interpretation. Poorly angulated radiographs are practically worthless. A series shows the various positions of the head of the condyle at various stages of opening the mouth.

extraoral exposures made with intraoral film

As we have seen, intraoral films may also be used extraorally. Usually the large occlusal film is used, but the smaller #2 film is also used. Extraoral radiographs of tooth structures are not as clear as intraoral exposures and fail to show many fine details. This, however, is of minor importance when one considers that limited access, gagging, or swelling might make it impossible to expose any films intraorally. Richard C. O'Brien in *Dental Radiography*[1] suggests several ways to make this exposure in areas of difficult third molar impactions, using occlusal film extraorally.

The following steps are suggested in making a survey of an impacted mandibular third molar area:

1. Adjust the ala-tragus line so that the occlusal plane of the maxillary arch is parallel to the plane of the floor.

2. Position the film extraorally, tube side toward the face, so that it is centered over the mandibular third molar area. Place the widest dimension of the film parallel with the lower border of the mandible and let the front edge of the film extend forward to the corner of the mouth.

3. Tell the patient to hold the film and to thrust the jaw forward to avoid superimposing the vertebrae over the site of the impaction.

4. Tilt the patient's head slightly toward the side of the film and direct the central ray toward the middle of the film at a vertical angulation of about minus 15 to 20 degrees through the point of entry on the side opposite the film, just below and behind the angle of the mandible. This enables the central ray to pass beneath the mandible without superimposing the structures of one side of the mandible on the other (Fig. 17–5).

5. Make this exposure with "D" speed film at 90 kVp, 10 mA, and 1/5 second, with the target-film distance from 15 to 18 inches.

1. O'Brien, Richard C. *Dental Radiography*, 2d ed. Philadelphia: W. B. Saunders Co., 1972.

A variation of this technique is suggested that shows both the maxillary and mandibular impacted third molar areas on the same film. Make two changes to accomplish this: (1) Position the film so that its longest dimension is vertical, its front edge extends to the corner of the mouth, and its lower border is even and parallel with the inferior border of the mandible, thus causing the occlusal plane between the maxillary and mandibular third molars to be at the center of the film; and (2) direct the central ray toward the center of the film at a vertical angulation of about minus 15 to 20 degrees through the point of entry on the side opposite to the film, about 1 inch above and 1/2 inch behind the angle of the mandible.

As this survey is primarily made to determine the location of the third molars rather than to evaluate the progress of decay, the dimensional distortion and magnification of the image from such an angulation do not detract from the diagnostic value of the radiograph.

panoramic radiography

Panoramic radiography enables the operator to produce an image of the entire dentition, the surrounding alveolar bone, the sinuses, and the temporomandibular joints on a single extraoral film. Instead of exposing 16 or more intraoral radiographs—a time consuming procedure—the entire exposure can be made in about 20 seconds. This makes

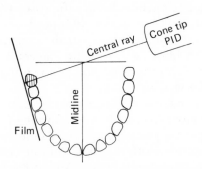

Fig. 17-5 Diagram indicating direction of the central ray (beam) and placement of the film and cone tip (PID) for the impacted third molar position. The occlusal film is placed with the widest dimension horizontally (long axis of film parallel to floor). Two changes are necessary to use this technique for the maxillary impacted third molar area. The film is placed vertically so that the upper half is centered over the maxillary third molar, and the center of the cone tip or PID is positioned approximately 1 inch above the angle of the mandible and just posterior border of the mandible. (From O'Brien, Richard C. *Dental Radiography*, 2d ed. Philadelphia: W. B. Saunders Co., 1972.)

the panoramic radiograph ideal for mass surveys, as are common in the military services, for children, for invalids, and for any situation where a rapid survey is desired. Many dentists make the routine full-mouth survey with a panoramic film and supplement it with four interproximal films, exposing periapical films only in areas where problems are suspected.

Panoramic radiography is a relatively new field which is still in the process of development. A number of foreign and domestic manufacturers produce panoramic x-ray machines, each of which differs from the others in size, appearance, and principles of operation. A few use an intraoral tube in which the target is at the end of a projection that is placed within the mouth and the film is placed inside a flexible cassette that is secured around the patient's face. Most panoramic machines have the tube on the outside. Usually the tube and the film rotate around the patient, but on some machines the patient and the film rotate while the tube remains fixed. This is known as curved surface *laminagraphy* (lamina meaning thin layer and graphy meaning to record), a technique by which various selected layers of body tissues can be studied a layer at a time.

In panoramic x-ray machines, the shape of the radiation beam is constricted to form a narrow band instead of the familiar cone shaped beam formed in the conventional x-ray machine. By using a narrow beam, one section only is exposed at a time—hence the name laminagraphy. A mechanism that moves the tube and the film in opposite directions simultaneously while the specific tissue layer remains in a fixed relationship to the tube and the film produces a clear image of the layer that is being examined, while at the same time blurring the adjacent tissues. This blurring of the other layers is necessary to prevent interference from the structures of the other layers that were not selected for viewing.

Changes are being made by the manufacturers so rapidly that it is not feasible to give more than a brief description of the best known panoramic machines. On one of these, the Panorex, the film is enclosed in a rigid cassette. Both the tube and film revolve around the seated patient as the exposure is made. An automatic lateral shifting of the chair in which the patient is sitting takes place midway through the cycle, producing the effect of two centers of rotation. This shift occurs as the tube passes behind the spinal column, and during this brief interval the machine automatically shuts down the milliamperage producing a blurred portion in the middle of the radiograph (Fig. 17–6). Since some structures are duplicated as a result of this shift, the central incisors being shown on both the right and left halves of the radiograph, some operators cut out the blurred and duplicating

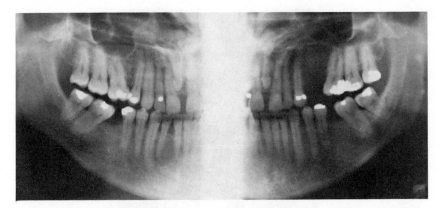

Fig. 17-6 Illustration of a large panoramic radiograph, showing effect of extractions on bone changes and tooth movement. The exposure was made with a Panorex machine. As with all extraoral films, a certain degree of magnification can be seen. The blurring in the center of the film and the duplication of tooth structures in the incisor regions is caused by the shift in position of the moving parts of the machine during the middle of the exposure. This, however, does not materially detract from the diagnostic quality of the radiograph.

area and fasten the remaining portions into the correct relationship. This makes it easier to view the radiograph.

On another panoramic machine, the Orthopantomograph, the film is contained in a flexible cassette adapted to a semicircular drum. The position of the patient does not change while three centers of rotation are used as the drum rotates around an axis and simultaneously from the patient's left side, around the front of his face, to his right side. Meanwhile the tube moves in the opposite direction, from the patient's right, around and behind his neck, and to his left side.

On still another panoramic machine, the Panelipse (Fig. 17–7), the film is enclosed in a flexible cassette which wraps around a circular drum. The position of the patient does not change as the tube head and the film travel in a continuously moving axis of rotation that describes an elliptical plane-in-focus. The size of the elliptical path is continuously variable so that the plane-in-focus will coincide with the dental arch of each patient. This results in the production of a continuous, non-interrupted image on the radiograph, and because the elliptical plane-in-focus adjusts to every patient's arch, such radiographs thus produced show a uniform magnification. Such magnification is an inherent feature of all panoramic radiographs.

Head positioning is very important in panoramic radiography, and some form of head positioning device must be used to keep the occlusal plane in proper relationship to the path of the tube head and

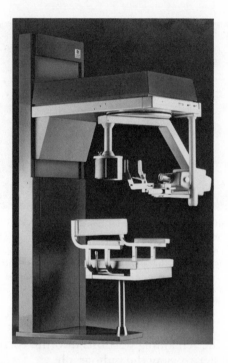

Fig. 17-7 Panelipse panoramic x-ray system. Produces a complete view of the entire oral region on one radiograph, with uniform magnification (19 percent) of all anatomy in the plane-in-focus. The overall length of the images are proportional to the actual lengths of each patient's dental arch. The exposure requires 20 seconds and the patient receives approximately 0.5 R during this interval. (Courtesy of General Electric Company.)

the film. One such head holder is shown in Figure 17-8. The complexity of the holders on different machines varies.

The procedures for making the exposures are similar on most panoramic machines. A brief sequence of operation would be:

1. Load the film into cassette. If the cassette is the flexible type it must also be attached to the drum. Identify the film.

2. Position the patient. Remove eyeglasses and removable appliances. On some units a locking pin must first be removed.

3. Make necessary adjustments to head holder and check profile index measurements. Select the proper kVp.

4. Depress the handswitch during the time of the exposure (20 to 22 seconds).

5. Deactivate the machine and release the patient. Remove cassette.

As the complexity of the controls and head holder adjustments varies from unit to unit, read the manufacturer's instructions carefully

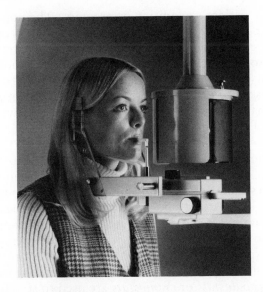

Fig. 17-8 Head positioner for panelipse panoramic system. Head holders and bite positioner centers and restrains patient. Automatically measures jaw size and allows operator to program the elliptical plane-in-focus to fit the arch size of each patient. Guide lines at both sides of the head allow accurate position of the ala-tragus line. Bite positioner insures proper alignment of anterior teeth and opens the bite to eliminate overlap of the occlusal surfaces. A direct reading size scale on the head positioner translates to the overhead jaw size setting scale. Infinite range of settings to accommodate all patients — from pedo to large adult. A wrap around film cassette with intensifying screens attaches firmly to the cassette holder drum. (Courtesy of General Electric Company.)

before attempting to operate an unfamiliar machine. If possible, have someone who is familiar with it give a demonstration. Although the panoramic x-ray machines are larger, costlier, and more complex than the conventional x-ray machines, their operation is much simpler and can be learned in less than an hour.

cephalometric radiography

Cephalometric headplates are extraoral radiographs of the head used for making skull and soft tissue measurements. Although requested occasionally by a general practitioner and more often by a prosthodontist, these are principally required by orthodontists and are an important part of the orthodontic diagnostic survey. Most modern orthodontists now require cephalometric headplates before treatment, at various stages of treatment, upon completion of treatment, and often as a follow-up procedure. Cephalometric tracings are made from these radiographs. It is now possible to feed the data and measurements derived from these tracings into computers for analysis of the patient's condition or progress. The importance of cephalometric radiography is increasing rapidly as more people than ever before are receiving orthodontic treatment. Therefore, dental auxiliary personnel should know something about exposure procedures and terms used to describe the basic anthropometric landmarks and planes inscribed on cephalometric tracings. *Anthropometry* is the science that deals with measurements of the size, weight, and proportions of the human body.

The word *cephalometric* means "having to do with the measurement of the head." A *cephalometer* is a device used to standardize the placement of the head during exposure. Either conventional x-ray machines modified for cephalometric work or special units may be used. The patient's head must be completely stable, as must the cassette that holds the film. In addition, a cephalometer allows the head to be positioned identically at different times, for a series of identical exposures. To do this, one coordinates the relationship between the direction of the PID, the patient, and the cassette. Devices called *cephalostats* or *craniostats* are used to stabilize the patient's head parallel to the film and at right angles to the direction of the beam of radiation. Ear rods are pushed into the external openings of the ear. These stabilize the head and also make it possible to secure the same position each time. The cassette with intensifying screens is aligned in a definite relationship to the cephalostats so that the patient's head is between it and the source of radiation. The PID is directed at 0-degrees angulation toward the patient and the film. On many special units it is possible to turn a knob and move the tube head up or down to correspond to the height of the cassette when the patient is seated in the chair. The target-film distance is normally 60 inches. Exposure time depends upon the type of film and intensifying screens used.

Cephalometric headplates may be either frontal (posteroanterior) or lateral skull projections (Fig. 17–9). Frontal headplates are especially indicated when asymmetry is suspected or a computer analysis is to be made. Because of their limited usefulness, frontal headplates are not part of the standard survey.

Lateral projections (centric soft tissue profiles) are frequently made, sometimes periodically throughout the treatment period. The centric soft tissue profile is used to determine the position of the jaws, the size of the jaws, the steepness of the angle of the mandible, and the relationship of the mandible and maxilla to each other. The profile of the nose, lips, and chin is an important consideration for the orthodontist because he must treat the face as well as the malocclusion. Lateral headplates are useful in determining if the malocclu-

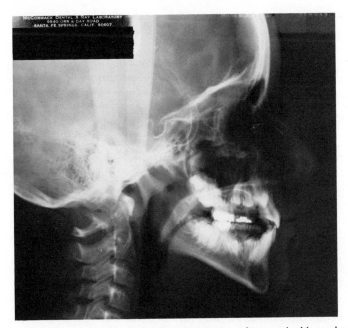

Fig. 17-9 Lateral skull cephalometric headplates are often required by orthodontists for making measurements of the head. Some form of device is essential to position the head to achieve standardization and to establish a fixed relationship between the x-ray tube, the patient's head, and the film cassette. Earplugs are used to stabilize and maintain the head position. For the lateral cephalometric headplate, the film is positioned in a plane parallel to the midsagittal plane of the patient and the central beam passes through both earplugs from a target-film distance of 60 inches or more. Cephalometric tracings may be made from these headplates to identify the positions of certain landmarks. (Courtesy of McCormack Dental X-Ray Laboratory.)

sion is (1) *dental*, involving only the teeth, (2) *skeletal*, with poor relationship of the maxilla and mandible, or (3) *skeletodental*, involving both teeth and jaw. Most malocclusions are of this type.

These projections may show soft tissues such as adenoidal or tonsilar tissues, aiding in the diagnosis of functional abnormalities such as mouth breathing. Blockage or obstruction of the airways by soft tissues may also contribute to abnormal tongue position.

Tracings of the centric soft tissue profile are made on acetate paper. A few of the more common landmarks and planes used are described below. The auxiliary working in an orthodontic practice should learn these terms as well as others not listed here. Some of these landmarks or planes are abbreviated; these abbreviations are shown in Figure 17-10.

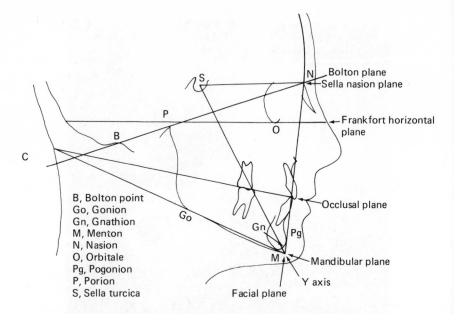

B, Bolton point
Go, Gonion
Gn, Gnathion
M, Menton
N, Nasion
O, Orbitale
Pg, Pogonion
P, Porion
S, Sella turcica

Fig. 17-10 Drawing from a cephalometric headplate showing some of the basic anthropometric landmarks. (From Wuehrmann, Arthur H., and Manson-Hing, Lincoln R. *Dental Radiology*, 2d ed. St. Louis: The C. V. Mosby Co., 1969. Used by the courtesy of Dr. J. Mehta and Dr. H. P. Hitchcock.)

cephalometric landmarks

A	*Subspinale*	The deepest point on the midline contour at the alveolar process between the anterior nasal spine and the prosthion—usually at the level of, and anterior to the apices of, the maxillary central incisors.
ANS	*Anterior Nasal Spine*	The most anterior point on the nasal floor of the nasal cavity.
B	*Bolton Point*	The highest point of the curvature at the notches behind the occipital condyles on the occipital bone.
Gn	*Gnathion*	The midpoint between the most anterior and inferior point on the bony chin (between pogonion and menton). It can be located by bisecting

		the facial plane and the mandibular plane.
Go	*Gonion*	The lowest posterior and most outward point on the angle of the mandible. It is located by bisecting the posterior ramal plane and the mandible plane angle.
M	*Menton*	The lowest point on the contour of the mandibular symphysis.
N	*Nasion*	The most anterior point of the nasofrontal suture on the midsagittal plane.
Or	*Orbitale*	The lowest point on the contour of the bony orbit.
P	*Porion*	The midpoint on the upper edge of the external auditory meatus (acoustic meatus).
Pg	*Pogonion*	The most anterior prominent point on the contour of the chin.
Pr	*Prosthion*	The alveolar point.
S	*Center Sella*	The center of the contour of the sella turcica—the pituitary fossa of the sphenoid bone.

cephalometric planes

Bolton Plane	The nasion to postcondylare plane. The line from the Bolton Point to the nasion.
Facial Plane	The line from the nasion to the pogonium.
Frankfort Plane	The horizontal plane between the porion and the orbitale.
Mandibular Plane	The line of the lower border of the mandible from the gonion to the menton.
Occlusal Plane	The plane between the maxillary and the mandibular teeth.

Posterior Ramal Plane   The posterior border of the ramus
of the mandible—a line from the
porion to the gonion.

For additional information on cephalometric landmarks and planes,
consult the various textbooks on orthodontia in the school library
or in the office.

Specific landmarks and their relationship to each other and to the
facial angle, the Frankfort plane, and the angle of convexity are measured from these cephalometric tracings. These measurements are then
compared to a group mean to determine the degree of deviation from
a pleasing facial pattern with excellent occlusion. This information
(often obtained through a computer) is then transferred to a graph
and included with the tracing and the headplate.

Most cephalometric headplates are exposed at professional radiography laboratories, because few orthodontic offices have the facilities
for exposing and developing them. Nor do they have ready access to
computers for ready analysis. Although some orthodontists have
trained personnel capable of making cephalometric tracings, most
do not. The auxiliary with such skills is in great demand.

bibliography

Crandell, Clifton E. *Dental Radiology for Auxiliary Personnel*,
Chapel Hill, N.C.: University of North Carolina Press, 1972.

Ennis, Leroy M., Berry, Harrison M., and Phillips, James E. *Dental
Roentgenology,* 6th ed. Philadelphia: Lea & Febiger, 1967.

O'Brien, Richard C. *Dental Radiography*, 2d ed. Philadelphia:
W. B. Saunders Co., 1972.

Wainwright, William Ward. *Dental Radiology*, New York: McGraw-
Hill Book Co., 1965.

Wuehrmann, Arthur H., and Manson-Hing, Lincoln R. *Dental
Radiology*, 2d ed. St. Louis: The C. V. Mosby Co., 1969.

X-Rays in Dentistry, Rochester, N.Y.: Eastman Kodak Co., 1972.

18

photography
in dental practice

importance of photography in dental practice

Modern cameras have made dental photography so simple that it is becoming a part of the standard routine in many dental offices. Photographs may be black and white or colored, prints or transparencies, rarely or frequently used in dentistry. In any case, dental auxiliaries usually do the photographic work. With a little practice most can produce good photographs. The normal procedure is to take photographs at the time of the examination and before dental work is started. Additional photographs may be taken to record some phase of restorative work in progress, and after treatment is completed. An orthodontist may desire periodic follow-up photographs.

Dental photographs have many uses; like radiographs, they become a part of the patient's record and can be used as evidence in court—an important consideration in these days of increasing malpractice suits. Such pictures also help insurance companies to settle claims resulting from accidental injuries to the teeth. Photographs are also used in patient education, including community dental health programs and presentations at clinics or lectures. They illustrate articles in publication, and serve as a means of identification.

The oral surgeon uses photography to demonstrate unusual surgical techniques; the orthodontist, for before-and-after studies to evaluate the success or failure of his treatment; the pedodontist, to alert the parent by showing him changes in the child's mouth; the endodontist, to demonstrate techniques and results; and the periodontist, to reassure the patient by demonstrating progress.

Most patients appreciate the thoroughness of the dentist who takes pictures. They can see their own dental conditions and observe progress. Most people want to improve their appearance and pictures can show them what has been done for others and what can be done for them. Likewise, pictures help people make up their minds about whether to undergo a specific treatment. Pictures also help the dentist keep the patient from expecting the impossible.

Dental photographs, like radiographs, may be either extraoral or intraoral. Extraoral photographs may be used to make profiles of the head or frontal views of the face. Intraoral photographs are used for closeups of the teeth, lesions inside the mouth, fractured teeth, cavity or crown preparations, and finished restorations.

types of cameras and lighting equipment

Cameras and lighting equipment suitable for dental photography vary from the fairly simple, relatively inexpensive equipment normally used to the complex and expensive apparatus used by research workers, clinicians, and lecturers.

The two most important items to the quality of the photographs are the lens and the lighting. The size and shape of the camera are relatively unimportant, because the principal functions of the camera body are to allow the operator to view the scene and control the exposure, and to house the film.

The cheapest cameras are the simplest; the expensive ones have many components and are complicated to operate. Most cameras suitable for dental photography fall somewhere in between. A typical camera has the following components: a film counter, a shutter-speed dial, a shutter release, a film-advance lever, a diaphragm ring, a distance scale, a lens, a rewind knob, a flash terminal, a viewfinder, a film pressure plate, film perforation sprockets, film take-up spool, and a film rewind button. Some of the last mentioned items are not found on cameras that use cartridge film. The instruction booklet that comes with the camera contains diagrams that show the location of the components and provides operational instructions.

The ideal camera for use in the dental office is the 35 mm. single lens reflex camera, which allows the object to be viewed directly through the lens. Such a camera, when special lenses, light attachments, and extension bellows are added, is extremely versatile and can be used for clinical as well as routine dental photography. However, this type of equipment is fairly complicated to assemble and use and requires a skilled photographer.

Lenses are the heart of any camera, and determine how much can be included in the photograph. There are standard, wide-angle, and telephoto lenses as well as special-purpose lenses. A fine lens will produce excellent details in all ranges for which it is designed, from closeup to distance. Most standard lenses are not suitable for distances less than three feet from the object. Dental photographs, even the frontal and profile views, are taken close up. Intraoral pictures are taken at 6 to 12 inches from the teeth.

Much easier to use are the fixed lens box type cameras and the instant process picture cameras in which the object is viewed through a rangefinder or a mirror system rather than directly through the lens. Both these types of camera, with the proper attachments, produce pictures that, though not of professional quality like those produced by the single lens reflex camera, are satisfactory for routine work. And a simple box camera can produce better pictures than an expensive one that is not set properly. A good rule in dental photography is to keep everything as simple as possible.

Several conversion kits are available that can be used to modify a number of good quality box cameras for closeup dental photography. One that is commonly used consists of a ringlight to provide the required illumination, a 45 mm. lens system capable of being rotated so that any one of four lenses can be positioned in front of the lens of the camera, and a series of different size metal locator frames. When these attachments are properly positioned, the operator has a choice of four lenses, each suitable for a different distance. The lenses and frames are color-coded to avoid confusion; the color in the circle around the lens must correspond to the color of the frame that is used. The smallest frame is used for extreme closeup photography, such as pictures of a crown or restoration; a slightly larger frame is used for taking a picture of an entire dental arch; a still larger frame is used for a frontal picture of all the teeth, as in the typical toothpaste advertising smile; and the largest frame is used for frontal or profile pictures. As the viewfinder of the camera is covered by these attachments it cannot be used; the frames allow the operator to see what area will appear on the finished picture. These cameras are easy to load, requiring only the insertion of a film cartridge. The camera is preset before the attachments are fastened to it, and no further focusing or changing of the controls is required.

Instant process picture cameras that require no focusing or exposure adjustments are available for dental use. Such cameras are handheld and have a built-in electronic flash (Fig. 18-1). A selection of basic camera parts, interchangeable lenses, and specialized clip-on accessories allows the user to assemble parts of his choice to make

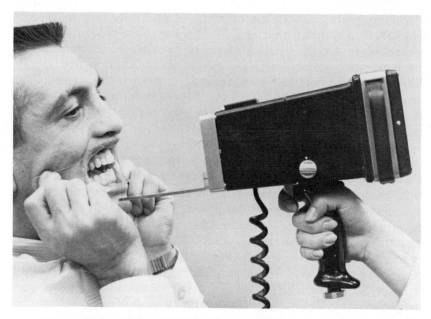

(a)

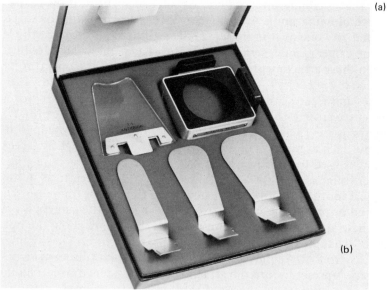

(b)

Fig. 18-1   Polaroid CU-5 land camera with attachments for intraoral photography. (a) Patient is holding cheek retractors for photograph of anterior teeth — either color or black and white; (b) attachments to fit on camera for life size (1:1) reproductions — other types attachments for one quarter life size (¼:1) and double life size (2:1) may be attached to this versatile camera which can be used for any type of instant intraoral or extraoral photography. (Courtesy of Polaroid Corporation.)

virtually every type of extraoral or intraoral picture—quarter size, life size, or double life size. Although lens and shutter settings can be changed manually, this is not necessary. A three-setting exposure program enables the photographer to adjust the setting according to the lens attached by flipping a switch on the camera.

To make a picture the camera is aimed at the object or the area to be photographed and the shutter release is triggered. Then two tabs are pulled from the back of the camera and the user waits for ten seconds for black and white film or one minute for color film. Pictures can be made in rapid succession because development takes place outside the camera.

A wide selection of films and accessories may be used in dental photography. Unless the films are desired for public presentation or the dentist's hobby is photography and he likes to use fancy equipment, the equipment should be kept simple to prevent errors. In most offices, where the auxiliaries take the photographs, equipment that requires little focusing or adjusting is preferred. If much photography is to be done, a professional versed in the art of photography should visit the dental office to advise on light conditions in the operatory, distances to be used, types of light, filters, and special colored backgrounds.

essentials of dental photography

Loading and unloading the cameras is becoming simpler all the time. The use of film cartridges, which are just dropped into the camera, eliminates the sometimes troublesome procedure of threading the film. Most cameras, when modified for dental use by attachments, use just one speed and not more than two apertures (lens openings). Therefore the operator has very little to do except to observe a few simple rules: (1) get as close to the subject as possible, (2) align the camera horizontally and vertically to straighten the picture, and (3) learn what the camera will take, thus avoiding *parallax*, a condition in which the viewing mechanism shows more than the taking lens; the photograph thus shows less than the photographer sees.

Good light is necessary in all dental photography. The light used varies with the complexity of the equipment and the amount of money the dentist is willing to invest in photographic equipment. Flashbulbs, incandescent light, or strobelights may be used. Best results in pictures can only be achieved with experience. An operator who cares about making good pictures will want to experiment with the effects of light, shadows, hair color, or skin tones. For example, the light from a pink floodlight kept 4 to 6 feet away from the face covers reflections on the skin and helps to minimize blemishes, or the placing of a colored background improves the contrast on a picture. Blondes are more difficult to photograph than brunettes; for best contrasts a dark background is used for blondes whereas a light background is used for brunettes.

Unless the camera is preset, as is the case with most fixed lens cameras modified for dental use, the operator must do three things: (1) focus the camera, (2) select the correct aperture or "f" stop, and (3) select the proper shutter speed.

On most cameras, one focuses by looking through the viewfinder or range finder and turning a ring or knob until the object appears sharp and definite.

The aperture and the shutter speed are synchronized to work together; thus the amount of light reaching the film is determined by a combination of the f stop and the shutter speed. A diaphragm behind the lens increases or decreases the opening through which light from the outside reaches the film, regulating the amount of light reaching the film. This opening is called the aperture or *f stop*. On most cameras, f stops range from f 2, which lets in a maximum of light, to f 22, which lets in a minimum. These f stops are usually marked on the dial that surrounds the lens as f 2, f 2.8, f 4, f 5.6, f 8, f 11, f 16, and f 22. Each larger number lets in half as much light as the preceding f stop (the amount of the light is determined by the inverse square law), provided that the exposure time is not changed. In dental photography, where concentrated artificial light is used, most extraoral exposures are made at f 16 and intraoral exposures at f 22. The reason for this is that less light is required when the camera is close and the light is concentrated inside the mouth and reflected by the linings of the cheeks. The camera and light are further away when the face or head is photographed and the light is diffused into the surrounding area.

As we have seen, the shutter speed also regulates the amount of light striking the film. The shutter is a halfmoon shaped piece of metal that opens or closes the aperture of the camera. Other shutters are made of black rubberized cloth with various-sized slits, or made of metal leaves. All accomplish the same function, to regulate the light by controlling the time of the exposure. On most cameras the shutter speed is expressed in fractions of a second, from 1/4 to 1/500 and less on sophisticated cameras. The lower the speed, the longer the shutter stays open. A speed of 1/125 second is recommended in dental photography. The use of a tripod to steady the camera is desirable whenever speeds less than 1/30 second are used—at which point "camera shake" becomes a problem.

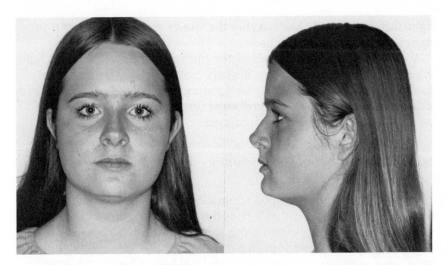

Fig. 18-2 Typical extraoral photographs used in dentistry. (a) Frontal view; (b) profile. (Courtesy of McCormack Dental X-Ray Laboratory.)

techniques for extraoral photography

Most dental photography is done with the patient sitting in the dental chair, although some dentists prefer to have the patient in a special room in which the photographic equipment can be set up permanently. In such a room, the walls are painted bluish or grayish to provide a better background.

Ask the patient to sit relaxed and still for profile and frontal pictures (Fig. 18-2). It is best to have men sit with the head straight; women's pictures are generally more pleasing if the head is tilted slightly. Always give women patients a chance to comb their hair first, because disarranged hair is always magnified in closeup photography.

Always point the camera slightly toward the patient and ask him to part his lips slightly. Because eye contact is essential to preserve personality, ask the patient to look forward at you but not at the light—looking at the light source causes a spot to appear on the pupil of the eye in the finished photograph; this spot is red on color photographs.

Artificial light is always required to produce good photographs. One can supplement the electronic flash on the camera with other lights placed in various positions. Side lighting hits the patient at a 90-degree angle; cross lighting helps to eliminate shadows; and back-lighting produces a pleasing effect in photographs of persons with

light skin and blonde hair. Avoid the use of front lighting, as it produces a shadow under the nose.

Wall colors affect the tones of the picture; white walls reflect light
whereas dark walls absorb it. Slightly tinted walls make the skin
look lighter. A more pleasing background can be provided by placing
a 3 by 4 ft. piece of tinted cardboard beside or behind the patient's
head. Light blue or gray is often used.

techniques for intraoral photography

Most intraoral photographs are made with the patient sitting in
the dental chair. The use of a tripod is generally not possible because
the camera must be held too close to the mouth. It is best to steady
yourself by placing one foot in front of the other in a bipod stance,
keep your arms close to the body, and hold your breath while press-
ing the plunger or trigger mechanism gently. Avoid the common mis-
take of blocking the lens opening with the finger or letting the
camera strap fall over it.

Use cheek retractors, mirrors, or tongue depressors in taking pictures of the back of the mouth. Two cheek retractors are needed to
pull the lips away so that one can take a picture showing all of the
front teeth (Fig. 18-3). It is always best to first ask the patient to
rinse his mouth to remove excess saliva, and then dry the areas of
interest with a gentle stream of warm air. If the patient cannot
manage to hold the cheek retractors, you may have to ask someone
else for assistance.

The flashgun or ringlight provides fairly even illumination. If additional light is available and desired, direct it from the side opposite
the side being photographed. Photograph mandibular teeth with the
camera and the attached light slightly above the occlusal plane, and
the maxillary teeth with the camera and the attached light slightly
below it. Tilt the patient's head in any direction that gives the best
lighting and access.

methods of identifying and filing
photographs and transparencies

All photographs and transparencies are a part of the patient's record. They are of little value, however, if they are not identified and
cannot be located when needed. Many workable systems of identification and filing have been devised. Prints are generally identified on
the back and placed in a special envelope on which the identifying

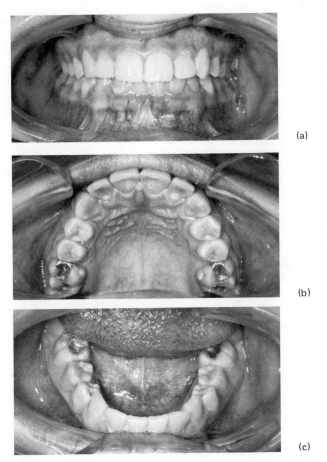

(a)

(b)

(c)

Fig. 18-3 Typical intraoral photographs. (a) Frontal view of occluded teeth;
(b) intraoral view of maxillary arch; (c) intraoral view of mandibular arch. (Courtesy of McCormack Dental X-Ray Laboratory.)

information is also marked. These envelopes may be attached to the
record card or filed separately.

Record the following data: the patient's name, the date of exposure, whether the picture is single or one of a series, its number in the
series, and the number of the file or drawer in which the envelope is
to be filed. Enter the file number on the record card to make it easier
to locate the picture.

Transparencies are normally kept in drawers or files with slots for
each slide. The margins of the transparencies may be used for identification. One system is to write the identification or file number
on the upper left corner, the patient's name on the lower left corner,
and the date on the lower right corner.

To reduce the danger of mixups or replacing pictures, view the prints or transparencies on the day they are returned from the processor and file them as soon as they are identified. Dental photography also requires record keeping. Record the identifying data not only on the envelope, but also on a daily log and on the record card. The data on the daily log includes the number of exposures made on each patient and whether these were intraoral or extraoral. If sophisticated equipment is used, record the type of film, shutter speed, lens opening, special lights, and so on.

Each office has its own code or system for recording data. Consecutive numbers may be used for newly photographed patients, letters to designate drawers in which the prints or transparencies are to be filed, numbers to indicate whether the picture is routine or comes under a special heading, such as periodontia, crown and bridge, prosthetics, or malocclusion. Such data are extremely valuable when one wants to locate examples of conditions to show a patient. Storing and indexing dental radiographs and transparencies is normally a duty of the dental assistant or receptionist.

More and more dentists are realizing the educational value and benefits of dental photography. With easy-to-operate cameras now available and improved photographic films, dental photography will become an integral part of dental practice in the future.

bibliography

Bruce, Helen Finn. *Your Guide to Photography*, New York: Barnes and Noble, 1965.

Chamberlain, Catherine. *An Introduction to the Science of Photography*, New York: The Macmillan Co., 1957.

Frehe, C. L. "Camera and Lighting Equipment in Dental Photography," *Indiana Journal of Medical Photography,* 1 (June 1965), 45–48.

Gibson, Lou H. "Electronic Flash for the Kodak Startech Camera," *Dental Radiography and Photography*, 38, No. 1 (1965), 16–21.

Gibson, Lou H. "Photography with the Dial-A-Matic Setup," *Dental Radiography and Photography*, 9, No. 2 (1966), 34–38.

Hein, John W. "Repeatable Serial Photography," *Dental Radiography and Photography*, 36, No. 1 (1963), 15–18.

La Cour, Marshall, and Lathrop, Irvin T. *Photo Technology*, Chicago: American Technical Society, 1967.

Mc Graham, William W. "Photography in Daily Practice," *Dental Radiography and Photography*, 38, No. 2 (1945), 39–42.

Sussman, Aaron. *The Amateur Photographer's Handbook*, New York: The Thomas Y. Crowell Company, 1962.

Wentworth, Edgar L. "Filing Color Slides in the Dental Office," *Dental Radiography and Photography*, 37, No. 2 (1964), 36–37.

19

patient education

patient education

One of the greatest services that the dental hygienist or assistant can render the patient is education. It is surprising how many patients, even today, do not understand radiography or its benefits. Many practitioners have not taken time to explain the advantages of routine radiographic examinations.

An effective method of patient education is to assemble a series of radiographs showing typical dental conditions, both normal and abnormal. Placed in convenient mounts, the radiographs are classified according to condition and shown to the patient on an illuminated viewer. Better yet—if facilities and projection equipment are available—radiographs can be placed in slide mounts and magnified on a wall or screen while the hygienist explains them. The auxiliary is well qualified to perform the role of educator. However, radiographs of persons other than the patient should always be used, because the law does not permit auxiliaries to interpret or diagnose radiographs.

benefits of preventive radiation

Everyone has heard about the bad effects of overexposure to radiation. Articles and pictures may frighten patients into avoiding all radiation. Radiographers should understand the hazards, but should educate patients about its benefits and the relative safety of dental radiation.

For one thing, a world without dental x-rays would be like a world without the automobile or the telephone. X-rays are a second pair of eyes to the dentist. Almost all modern dental techniques would be unworkable without radiation. Patients would suffer unnecessary pain if the dentist could not locate the source of their trouble. Radiographs prevent unnecessary removal of teeth, allow diagnosing conditions in early stages, when they can be treated, and even save lives by disclosing malignancies.

Moreover, the auxiliary can reassure the patients about radiation safety. Modern x-ray machines are designed for safety. The use of electronic timers and high-speed film has reduced the amount of radiation from a full-mouth exposure to a fraction of that formerly produced in a single exposure.

conclusion

Dental patients are not the only ones who benefit from the controlled use of radiation in the dental practice. Non-patients also benefit from radiographs shown at community health centers, P.T.A. meetings, schools, or dental health meetings or lectures. They learn certain conditions can only be discovered in time to correct them if radiographs are taken, and may thus be convinced to visit the dentist.

Some conditions that radiographs can demonstrate are periodontal changes and other pathological conditions associated with the loss of bone structures, the damage that can be caused by submarginal and proximal calculus deposits, the effect on the occlusion caused by premature loss or the prolonged retention of the deciduous teeth, the presence of unerupted or supernumerary teeth, the effect of losing the permanent teeth and the importance of having replacements, and the extent or presence of carious lesions not visible to the eye.

Of course, the benefits of radiography depend upon the radiograph's diagnostic quality. Each step in the process, though small, can be significant. A little error at any step can be compounded by others until it ruins the results. To obtain a good radiograph, one must pay meticulous attention to all phases of exposure technique, and keep the processing area clean.

Every operator of x-ray equipment should try to achieve perfection with each radiograph. The operator who takes pride in his work, constantly reviews techniques, and keeps up with the latest methods by reading books and professional articles, and attending lectures and seminars enhances his own professional status. Most important, he benefits the patient and dentistry by rendering the finest possible preventive service.

bibliography

Ennis, Leroy M., Berry, Harrison M., and Phillips, James E. *Dental Roentgenology*, 6th ed. Philadelphia: Lea & Febiger, 1967.

Wainwright, William Ward. *Dental Radiology*, New York: McGraw-Hill Book Co., 1965.

Wuehrmann, Arthur H., and Manson-Hing, Lincoln R. *Dental Radiology*, 2d ed. St. Louis: The C. V. Mosby Co., 1969.

glossary

This glossary includes not only terms used in the text and student workbook, but also terms frequently encountered in other publications on radiography. The student is encouraged to consult these as supplementary reading. Definitions may vary slightly from source to source. The use of a medical dictionary is also recommended.

Absorbed Dose: The energy imparted to matter by ionizing particles per unit of mass of irradiated material at the place of interest. The special unit of absorbed dose is the *rad*.

Absorption: The process through which radiation imparts some or all of its energy to any material through which it passes.

Acidifier: A chemical (acetic acid) in the fixer solution that neutralizes the alkali in the developer solution and stops further action of the developer.

Activator: A chemical (usually sodium carbonate) in the developer solution that causes the emulsion on the radiographic film to swell and initiates the reducing action of the developing agents. This sodium carbonate makes the developer alkaline.

Acute: Having a rapid onset, short severe course, and pronounced symptoms; opposite to chronic.

Acute Radiation Syndrome: Symptoms of the short-term radiation effects after a massive dose of ionizing radiation.

Added Filtration: Added to the inherent filtration built into the x-ray machine. This added filtration is in the form of thin disks of pure aluminum, which can be inserted between the x-ray tube and the lead collimeter when the inherent filtration is not sufficient to meet modern radiation safety requirements. The added filtration absorbs some of the longer, useless wavelengths and prevents their passage through the patient's tissues.

Adumbration: The production of a fuzzy shadow around the images on the radiograph.

Alkalizer: (See **Activator**.)

Alpha Particle: A common form of particulate (corpuscular) radiation. Alpha particles contain two protons and two neutrons and are positively charged. Symbol α (Greek lower case alpha).

Alternating Current: Electric current that changes its direction of flow 60 times per second. As it changes direction twice in each full cycle, there is a change every 1/120 second. Alternating current is used in most x-ray machines in the United States.

Aluminum Equivalence: The thickness of aluminum affording the same degree of attenuation, under specified conditions, as the material in question.

Amperes: Electric quantity or amount of electric current flowing through an electrical circuit.

Angstrom Unit: A unit of measurement that describes the wavelengths of certain high frequency radiations. One Angstrom unit (A.U. or Å) measures 1/100,000,000 of a centimeter. Most wavelengths used in dentistry vary from about 0.1 A.U. to a maximum of 1.0 A.U.

Angulation: The direction in which the central rays and the PID of the x-ray machine is directed toward the teeth and the film. (See **Horizontal Angulation, Negative Angulation, Positive Angulation, Vertical Angulation,** and **Zero Angulation.**)

Anode: The positive electrode (terminal) in the x-ray tube. Although the anode alternately changes from positive to negative, x-rays can only be produced during the phase of the alternating current cycle when the anode is positive. This is a tungsten block, normally set at a 20-degree angle facing the cathode, imbedded in the copper portion of the terminal. The roentgen rays emanate from the point of impact of the electronic stream (cathode rays) from the cathode.

Anterior Nasal Spine (ANS): The most anterior point on the floor of the nasal cavity. This is located at the midsagittal plane.

Anthropometry: The science that deals with the measurement of the size, weight, and proportions of the body. Anthropometric landmarks and planes are inscribed on cephalometric tracings used by orthodontists.

Aperture: An opening in the tube head that is covered with a permanent seal of glass, beryllium, or aluminum through which the x-rays leave the tube head. The aperture is opposite the window in the x-ray tube and is the place where the PID attaches to the tube head. It is also called the *port*.

Area Monitoring: The routine monitoring of the level of radiation in an area such as a room, building, space around radiation emitting equipment, or outdoor space.

Atom: The smallest particle of an element that has the properties of that element. Atoms are extremely minute and are made up of a number of subatomic particles. (See **Protons, Electrons,** and **Neutrons.**)

Attenuation: In radiography, the process by which a beam of radiation is reduced in energy when passing through matter. Lead is most often used to absorb and stop the passage of undesirable radiation.

Autotransformer: A voltage compensator that corrects minor fluctuations in the current flowing through the x-ray machine. A metal core wound with a single coil and located in the tube head.

Background Radiation: Ionizing radiation that is always present. It consists of cosmic rays from outer space, naturally occurring radiation from the earth and materials around us, and radiation from radioactive materials.

Backscatter: Radiation that is deflected by scattering processes at angles greater than 90 degrees to the original direction of the beam of radiation.

Beta Particle: A form of particulate radiation. High-speed negative electrons. Symbol β (Greek lower case beta).

Binding Energy: The internal energy within the atom that holds its components together.

Bisecting Technique (Bisecting-Angle or Short Cone Technique): An exposure technique in which the central beam of radiation is directed perpendicularly toward an imaginary line which bisects the angle formed by the recording plane of the film and the long axis of the tooth.

Bisector: The imaginary line that bisects the angle formed by the film and tooth. (See **Bisecting Technique**.)

Bitetab (Bitewing Tab): A piece of heavy paper or linen and paper that is attached at the center of the film packet and on which the patient bites to stabilize the film during an interproximal (bitewing) exposure.

Bitewing Radiograph: A radiograph that shows the crowns of both the upper and lower teeth on the same film. (See **Interproximal Radiograph**.)

Bolton Plane: A plane used in cephalometric radiography denoting a line from the Bolton Point to the nasion.

Bolton Point: A term used in cephalometric radiography denoting the highest point of curvature at the notches behind the occipital condyles.

Bremsstrahlung: German, meaning "braking radiation." The stopping or slowing of the electrons of the cathode stream as they collide with the nuclei of the target atoms.

Cassette: A rigid film holder consisting of a case with a hinged lid, each with an intensifying screen. Most cassettes are for use with extraoral films.

Cathode: The negative electrode (terminal) in the x-ray tube. Although the anode alternately changes from negative to positive, the electrons of the cathode stream flow to the anode to produce x-rays only when the cathode is in the negative phase of the alternating current cycle. The cathode consists of a tungsten filament wire that is set in a molybdenum focusing cup that directs the cathode stream toward the target on the anode.

Cathode Stream (Beam or Ray): The stream of electrons traveling from the heated filament of the cathode toward the target on the anode inside the x-ray tube. This beam of electrons travels at approximately half the speed of light. The speed depends upon the electromotive force (kilovoltage) that is applied.

Center Sella: A term used in cephalometric radiography to denote the center of the contour of the sella turcica on the sphenoid bone.

Central Beam (Ray): The central portion of the primary beam of radiation.

Cephalometer: A headholder or precision instrument used to stabilize the patient's head during exposure. This usually has cephalostats or craniostats, devices used to standardize the procedure so that identical results may be obtained each time. This holds the head parallel to the film and at right angles to the radiation beam.

Cephalometric Radiographs (Headplates): Lateral and posteroanterior extraoral head films. Much used in orthodontic treatment, they are used less often in prosthodontic treatment.

Cephalometric Tracings: Tracings from a cephalometric headplate made on acetate. These tracings indicate the location of various planes and points of interest to the orthodontist. Not all tracings show the same planes or points. The data are used to measure existing conditions and compare them with future or desirable conditions.

Characteristic Radiation: A form of radiation produced when the electrons of the cathode stream collide with the electrons in the energy levels of the target atom with sufficient force to remove them from that energy level. When that happens, the expelled electron is replaced by an electron from the next outer level, and this electron takes on the characteristics of the one that was removed by the collision.

Chromosomes: Structures found in the cell nuclei, which carry the hereditary materials. These are constant in number for each species. The chromosomes are adversely affected by radiation exposure; therefore protective lead aprons are used to protect the gonadal areas.

Collimation: The restriction of the useful beam to an appropriate size; generally, to a diameter of 2¾ inches at the skin surface.

Collimator: A diaphragm or tubular device, usually lead, designed to restrict the dimensions of the useful beam.

Cone (PID): A cone or cylindrical position indicating device (PID) to indicate the direction of the central beam of radiation. The length of the cone helps to establish the desired target-surface distance.

Cone Cut: A term used to describe a technique error in which the central beam is not directed toward the center of the film. This produces a blank area in that part of the radiograph that was not reached by the radiation.

Contrast: The visual differences between shades ranging from black to white in adjacent areas of the radiographic film. A radiograph that shows few shades is said to have short-scale contrast, while one that shows many variations in shade is said to possess long-scale contrast. Generally, the use of increased kilovoltage results in the production of a radiograph with long-scale contrast.

Control Panel: That portion of the x-ray machine which houses the major controls.

Controlled Area: A defined area in which the occupational exposure of personnel to radiation is under the supervision of the radiation protection supervisor. The dental office is designated as a controlled area: a public hallway or traffic corridor through a dental office is not so considered if used by the public.

Corpuscular Radiation: Minute subatomic structures such as protons, electrons, neutrons, and alpha, beta, and gamma particles of radiation. These particles occupy space, have mass and weight, and, with the exception of neutrons, have an electrical charge.

Crest: In radiation, the peak of an electromagnetic wave. The distance from crest to crest determines the wavelengths, hence its penetration ability.

Cross-Sectional Technique: A technique used in occlusal radiography, in which the central ray is directed toward the area of interest and parallel to the long axes of the teeth and adjacent areas.

Current: In radiation, a flow of electricity from a point of higher potential to a point of lower potential. The electric current used in most homes and dental offices is spoken of as "line current."

Cutting Reducer: A chemical used to lighten a radiograph that has been accidentally overexposed or overdeveloped. The chemical removes layer after layer of the metallic silver on the radiograph until the desired density is produced.

Deadman Switch: A switch so constructed that a circuit closing contact can only be maintained by continuous pressure by the operator.

Decay Process: In radiography, the radioactive disintegration of the nucleus of an unstable element by the emission of particles, photons of energy, or both.

Definition: In radiography, the sharpness and clarity of the outline of the structures on the image shown on the film. Poor definition is generally caused by movement of the patient, film, or the tube head during exposure.

Density: In radiography, film blackening (the amount of light transmitted through a film). The simplest way to increase or decrease the density of a radiograph is to increase or decrease the milliamperage and exposure time (milliampere/seconds).

Depth Dose: The total amount of radiation at any given point inside the patient or object. This is generally estimated by measuring the radiation first at the point of entry and then at the point of exit.

Detail: The point by point delineation of the minute structures visible in the shadow images on the radiograph. Detail may be good or poor. The best method of controlling detail is through selecting the best kilovoltage for the desired result and through careful processing.

Developer: The chemical solution used in film process that makes the latent image visible.

Developer Agent: Elon and hydroquinone, substances that reduce the halides in the film emulsion to metallic silver. Elon brings out the details and hydroquinone brings out the contrast in the film.

Dexter: (See **Phantom.**)

Diaphragm: A plate, usually lead, with a central aperture so placed as to restrict the useful beam. (See **Collimator.**)

Direct Current: - Electric current that flows continuously in one direction. Unidirectional current is produced in batteries but can not be used in x-ray machines unless they are modified.

Dispenser: In radiography, a lead-lined chute or container from which unexposed film packets can be removed one at a time.

Dosage: The radiation delivered to a specified area of the body measured in roentgen units. The dosage may be measured in air or at the skin surface.

Dose: The total amount (quantity) of radiation in roentgens at any given point, measured in air (that is, in the radiation field without the presence of the human body). Measurements inside the body are difficult, if not impossible, to make. Doses are often spoken of as absorbed, depth, entrance, exposure, erythema, skin, or surface doses.

Dose Equivalent: A quantity used for radiation protection purposes that expresses on a common scale for all radiations the irradiation incurred by exposed persons. It is defined as the product of absorbed dose in rads and certain modifying factors. The unit of dose equivalent is the *rem*.

Dose Rate: The radiation dose received per unit of time.

Dosimeter: A small device, usually the size of a fountain pen, used to measure an accumulated dose of radiation. This device contains a small ionizing chamber and an electrometer that can be read by the person wearing the dosimeter.

Electrode: Either of two terminals of an electric source; in the x-ray tube, either the anode or the cathode.

Electromagnetic Radiation: Forms of energy propelled by wave motion as photons of energy. This is a combination of electric and magnetic energy. This radiation has no charge, mass, or weight, and travels at the speed of light. These forms of energy differ tremendously in wavelength, frequency, and properties. For convenience they are arranged in diagrammatic form as the electromagnetic spectrum.

Electromagnetic Spectrum: Types of electromagnetic energies arranged in diagrammatic form on a chart. These include radio and television waves, infrared waves, visible light, ultraviolet waves, roentgen (x-rays), gamma rays, and cosmic radiations. The longer wavelengths are measured in meters and the shorter ones in Angstrom units.

Electromotive Force: The difference in potential between the cathode and the anode in the x-ray tube (generally expressed in kilovolts).

Electron: A negatively charged particle of the atom containing much energy and little mass.

Electron Cloud: A mass of free electrons that hovers around the filament wire of the cathode when it is heated to incandescence. The number of free electrons increases as the filament heat becomes greater. These free electrons become the cathode stream when the high-voltage circuit in the x-ray tube is activated.

Electron Shells: (See **Energy Levels.**)

Elongation: A term used in radiography to refer to a distortion of the image in which the tooth structures appear longer than the anatomical size. This is most often caused by insufficient vertical angulation of the central beam.

Emulsion: The coating on radiographic film, a gelatinous solution containing silver halides.

Emulsion Speed: The sensitivity of the film to the radiation exposure.

Energy: In physics, the ability to do work and overcome resistance. In radiography, the force that propels the electrons or the power of the wavelengths that enables them to penetrate the materials in their path.

Energy Levels (Electron Shells or Orbits): A term used in chemistry and physics to denote spherical layers or levels containing the electrons of the atom. The simplest atom has but one energy level. The more complex atoms have many energy levels.

Enhancement: Intensification of detail, making a radiograph easier to interpret.

Enhancer: A device that brings out details on a radiograph. Contains focusing devices and magnifying lenses.

Entrance Dose (Exposure Dose or Skin Dose): Radiation dosage at the point where it enters the patient.

Erythema Dose (Erythema Exposure): Radiation overdose that produces temporary redness of the skin. This condition becomes visible when the patient receives about 25 roentgens and will generally disappear in a short time if no further radiation is received.

Exit Dose: The amount of exposure received at that point where the beam of radiation exits from the patient.

Exposure: A measure of ionization produced in air by gamma or x-radiation. It is the sum of the electrical charges of all of the ions of one sign produced in air when all electrons liberated by photons in a volume element of air are completely stopped in air, divided by the mass of air in the volume present. The special unit of exposure is the roentgen. For radiation protection purposes, the number of roentgens may generally be considered to be numerically equivalent to the number of *rads* or *rems*.

Exposure Holder: Two pieces of cardboard that are hinged on one end and have a metal clasp on the other end to tightly lock the holder after an extraoral film is inserted into a paper envelope within the holder. Used to make extraoral exposures.

Exposure Rate: The exposure per unit of time.

Extension Arm: A flexible arm from which the tube head is suspended.

Extension Cone (Extension Tube): A long cone or tube-shaped positioning indicating device.

Extraoral: Outside the mouth.

"f" Stop: A term used in photography to describe the size of the lens aperture.

Facial Plane: A term used in cephalometric radiography. The line from the nasion to the pogonium.

Farmer's Solution: A chemical reducer used to lighten a dark overexposed or overdeveloped film.

Filament: The spiral tungsten coil in the focusing cup of the cathode of the x-ray tube.

Film Badge: A device containing a special type of film, worn by persons frequently exposed to radiation. When properly developed and interpreted, it gives an accurate measurement of the exposure received during the time the badge was worn.

Film Holder: A mechanical device used to hold and stabilize dental x-ray film in the mouth.

Film Packet: The intraoral film that is wrapped and enclosed for dental use by the manufacturer. It contains one or two films, a dark protective paper on either side, a thin sheet of lead foil on the back side of the film, and a semi-moisture proof outer wrap.

Film Safe: A lead-lined receptable for storing exposed dental film packets.

Film Sensitivity: (See **Emulsion Speed.**)

Filter: Absorbing material, usually aluminum, placed in the path of the beam of radiation to remove the more absorbable components (the undesired longer wavelengths).

Filtration: The use of absorbers for selectively attenuating or screening out the low-energy x-ray photons from the primary beam. (See **Added Filtration, Inherent Filtration,** and **Total Filtration.**)

Fixer: In radiography or photography, a solution of chemicals that stops the action of the developer and makes the image permanently visible.

Fixing Agent: Sodium thyosulfate, also known as "hypo" or hyposulfite of sodium. It is one of several chemical ingredients of the fixer solution and functions to remove all unexposed and any remaining undeveloped silver bromide grains from the emulsion.

Fluorescence: The emission of a glowing light by certain mineral salts when they are struck by particular wavelengths. In radiography, the calcium tungstate that is in the emulsion of the intensifying screen of cassettes glows and gives off a bluish light when the crystals are struck by the x-ray photons.

Focal Spot: A small area on the target on the anode toward which the electrons from the focusing cup of the cathode are directed. X-radiation originates at the focal spot.

Focusing Cup: A curved depression in the face of the cathode that contains the tungsten filament. This depression is cuplike in shape and designed to project the free electrons toward the tungsten target of the anode.

Fog: A cloudy appearance of the finished radiograph caused by any of several factors such as old or contaminated processing solutions, exposure to chemical fumes, faulty safelight, or scatter radiation.

Foreshortening: A term used in radiation to refer to a distortion of the image in which the tooth structures appear shorter than their actual anatomic size. This is most often caused by excessive vertical angulation of the central beam.

Frequency: The number of crests of a wavelength passing a given point per second. This provides an indication of the energy of the radiation. The higher the frequency, the shorter the wavelength. The shortest wavelengths have the most energy and penetrating ability.

Full-Mouth Survey: The complete radiographic examination of the mouth in which a film is positioned periapically in each major tooth area. This normally entails a minimum of 14 films. Often over 20 films. Generally such a survey also includes interproximal films.

Gamma Rays: A form of electromagnetic radiations similar to x-rays but shorter in wavelength. Usually produced spontaneously in the form of emission from radioactive substances.

Geiger Counter: A form of radiation monitoring device that counts the ionizing particles that pass through it. A needlelike electrode inside a gas filled chamber sets up a current in an electric field whenever the gas is ionized by radiation.

Genes: The fundamental units of inheritance, arranged on the chromosomes and carrying the individual traits of the organisms.

Genetic Cells: The cells contained within the testes and ovaries, containing the genes.

Genetic Effects: Radiation effects upon the genes and hence on future generations. It is believed that massive exposure of the genes to radiation may produce mutations.

Geometric Unsharpness: An inherent property of the focal spot that causes the production of double images and poor definition on the radiograph. Particularly when there is motion of the tube head, such secondary shadows will surround the primary shadows of the image.

Gnathion (Gn): In cephalometric radiography, the midpoint between the most anterior and inferior point on the bony chin between the pogonion and menton.

Gonion (Go): A term used in cephalometric radiography to describe the lowest, posterior, and most outward point on the angle of the mandible.

Grenz Rays: The longest of the x-rays, known as soft radiation because they have little penetrating power. Utilized in industry but of no dental value.

Half Life: The period required for the disintegration of half of the atoms in a sample of some specific radioactive substance.

Half-Value Layer: The thickness of a specified substance that, when introduced into the path of a given beam of radiation, reduces the exposure rate by half.

Halide: A compound of a halogen (astatine, bromine, chlorine, fluorine, or iodine) with another element or radical. In radiography a halide, usually bromide of silver, is suspended in the gelatin that coats the film base.

Hardening Agent (Hardener): Potassium alum, one of the chemicals of the fixing solution. It functions to shrink and harden the wet emulsion.

Hard Radiation: Rays of high energy and extremely short wavelengths. Essential for dental radiography.

High-Voltage Transformer (Step-Up Transformer): A device consisting of two metal cores and coils so positioned within the circuitry of the tube head that it is capable of increasing the potential of the line current to the high kilovoltage that is required to produce x-radiation.

Horizontal Angulation: The direction of the central beam in a horizontal plane. Faulty horizontal angulation is the main cause of overlapping the proximal structures during exposure.

Identification Dot: A small circular embossed mark on the corner of each x-ray film. The raised side of this convexity is always placed toward the side facing the x-ray beam. The identification dot makes it possible to determine whether the exposure was made on the patient's right or left side.

Image: In radiography, the duplicate in outline form of the structures exposed to radiation. A latent (invisible) image forms on the film when it is exposed. This latent image becomes visible after development and final processing.

Incandescence: In radiography, the stage in which the tungsten filament in the cathode becomes red-hot with heat and glows, thus liberating free electrons that swarm around the glowing wire to form the electron cloud.

Inherent Filtration: The filtration placed in the x-ray tube by the manufacturer. This includes the glass x-ray tube envelope, the insulating materials of the tube and tube head, and the materials that seal the port or aperture.

Intensifying Screens: A card or plastic sheet coated with calcium tungstate or similar fluorescent salt crystals, and positioned in the cassette so that it contacts the film. When exposed to radiation, the fluorescent salts glow, giving off a bluish light that along with the radiation causes the latent image to form faster than is possible when radiation only is used.

Interproximal Radiograph (Bitewing Radiograph): A radiograph that shows the crowns of both the upper and lower teeth on the same film. (See **Bitewing Radiograph**.)

Intraoral: Inside the mouth.

Intraoral Cassette: A very small cassette holding an occlusal film. Its purpose is to reduce exposure time through the action of the intensifying screens.

Intraoral Radiograph: A radiograph produced when the film is placed within the mouth and exposed.

Inverse Square Law: A rule stating that the intensity of radiation is inversely proportionate to the squares of the distances measured from the source of the radiation to the point of measurement. Thus, as distances are increased, radiation intensity at the object is decreased, and vice versa. This principle is used to determine target-film distance or the relative increase or decrease in radiation that a person receives at a given distance from the source.

Ion: An electrically charged particle from an atom or a molecule.

Ionization: The change that takes place within an atom when the electrons are gained or lost and the atom loses its neutrality, becoming positively or negatively charged.

Ionizing Chamber: A cylinder or enclosure in a monitoring device that contains electrodes. An electric field is maintained between them for the purpose of collecting the charge when the gas or air in the chamber is ionized during exposure to radiation.

Ionizing Radiation: Radiation that is capable of producing ions in the tissues exposed to it. Such a separation of the electrons from the tissue atoms and molecules is believed to produce undesirable biologic changes in some body tissues.

Irradiation: The exposure of an object or a person to radiation. This term can be applied to radiations of various wavelengths, such as infrared rays, ultraviolet rays, x-rays, and gamma rays.

Isotope: An alternate form of an element, having the same number of protons but a different number of neutrons inside the nucleus. Elements may have several forms of isotopes. Many isotopes are radioactive.

Kilovolt (kV): A unit of electromotive force, equal to 1000 volts, that drives the electric current through the circuit. High kilovoltage is essential for the production of dental x-rays.

Kilovolt Peak (kVp): The crest value in kilovolts of the potential difference of a pulsating potential generator. When only half the wave is used, the value refers to the useful half of the cycle.

Kinetic Energy: The power or potential force of atoms that are constantly in motion.

Laminagraphy: A technique used in some forms of panoramic radiography that makes a record of one section of the exposed tissues at a time (lamina meaning thin layer and graphy meaning to record).

Latent Image: The invisible image produced when the film is exposed to the x-ray photons. This image remains invisible until the film is processed.

Latent Period: The time between exposure to radiation and the first clinically observable symptoms.

Lateral Headplate (Lateral Radiograph): Large extraoral film placed against either side of the head and parallel to it. Used extensively in cephalometric radiography.

Lateral Jaw Survey: An extraoral exposure of either side of the patient's face that produces an image of both the maxilla and mandible on the same film.

Lead Equivalence: The thickness of a material that affords the same degree of attenuation to radiation as a specified thickness of lead.

Lead Protective Apron: Apron made of lead or lead- equivalent materials. These cover the patient's gonadal areas to protect them from radiation.

Leakage Radiation: A form of radiation that bounces off the target inside the tube and escapes out of the tube head at places other than the aperture.

Light Fog: Clouding or darkening of radiographic film through accidental exposure to bright light or prolonged exposure to a safelight.

Line Current: The electric current normally passing through the electric lines in most homes and offices. In the United States, this is generally a 110-volt alternating current.

Line Focus Principle: The method by which the size of the focal spot is reduced to the desired size by the manufacturer. By facing the target at an angle toward the cathode filament, the electron beam is focused into a narrow rectangle on the anode. When viewed from below, as from the position of the film packet, the rectangular area looks like a small square.

Line Switch: The toggle switch that is used to turn the x-ray machine on or off.

Long-Scale Contrast: The variations in contrast, with many shades of gray, shown on radiographs exposed with high kilovoltage.

Low-Voltage Transformer (Step-Down Transformer): A device consisting of two metal cores and coils so positioned within the circuitry of the tube head that it is capable of decreasing the line voltage to between 3 and 12 volts. Such voltage is required in the cathode to warm up the filament wire.

Maximum Permissible Accumulated Exposure: The maximum accumulated exposure that a person who is occupationally exposed may have at any given time of his life. This is determined by the formula 5 (N minus 18) where N equals the individual's age at his last birthday.

Maximum Permissible Dose Equivalent (MPDE): For radiation purposes, the maximum dose equivalent that a person or body part is allowed to receive in a stated period of time. It is the dose of ionizing radiation that, in the light of present knowledge, is not expected to cause detectable body damage to the average person at any time during his lifetime. For whole-body radiation this is currently established at 5 rems per year for radiation workers.

Maximum Permissible Dose Rate (MPDR): The maximum rate at which occupationally exposed persons may be exposed to x-radiation.

Menton (Me): A term used in cephalometric radiography to describe the lowest point on the contour of the mandibular symphysis.

Midsagittal Plane (Midsagittal Line): An imaginary vertical line or plane passing through the center of the body that divides it into a right and left half.

Milliammeter: A device on the control panel of many x-ray machines for determining and controlling the number of milliamperes of electric current flowing through.

Milliampere (mA): The milliampere is one-thousandth of an ampere. In radiography, the milliamperage determines the number of x-ray photons that are produced. (See **Ampere**.)

Milliampere/Second (mAs): The relationship between the milliamperage used and the exposure time in seconds. When one is increased, the other must be correspondingly decreased if the density of the exposed radiograph is to remain the same.

Milliroentgen (mR): One-thousandth of a roentgen.

Molecule: A chemical combination of two or more atoms that forms the smallest particle of a substance that retains the properties of that substance. The breaking up of any molecule into its constituent atoms changes its character.

Monitoring: In radiation, the use of any of several devices to determine whether an area is within safe radiation limits or whether a person's exposure is within permissible limits. (See **Area Monitoring** and **Personnel Monitoring**.)

Mutation: A change in the hereditary pattern of an organism. The change itself, if the organism survives, becomes hereditary. It is currently believed that any radiation exposure to the reproductive cells is capable of causing some form of mutation.

Nasion (N): In cephalometric radiography, the most anterior point of the naso frontal suture on the midsagittal plane.

Negative: A photographic or radiographic film wherein light and dark areas of the subject are shown in reverse.

Negative Angulation (Negative Vertical Angulation or Minus Angulation): Angulation achieved by pointing the tip or end of the PID upward from a horizontal plane. In the bisecting technique, negative angulation is used to make all mandibular exposures.

Negative Ion: An ion that has a negative electric charge. (See **Ion**.)

Neutron: One form of corpuscular radiation (particulate), or subatomic particle consisting of a combination of a proton and electron. A neutron has no electric charge and has about the same mass as a proton.

Non-Screen Film (No-Screen Film): A form of extraoral film that has an extra-thick coating of emulsion and is sensitive to radiation only when used inside an exposure holder. (See **Screen Film**.)

Object: In dental radiography, whatever is being radiographed, usually a tooth or teeth.

Occlusal Radiographs: Radiographs produced by placing the film along the incisal or occlusal plane and having the patient stabilize it by biting down on it. In addition to the teeth, occlusal radiographs may show surrounding maxillary or mandibular bone structures. Depending on the film placement and angle of exposure, cross-sectional or topographic radiographs are produced. (See **Cross-Sectional Technique** and **Topographical Technique**.)

Operator (Radiographer): The person operating any x-ray equipment to make exposures. A radiographer.

Oral Radiographic Survey: An examination of the teeth based on one or more radiographs of the dental area of interest.

Oral Radiography: All the procedures needed to produce radiographs of the teeth or head. These include adjustments of the x-ray machine, preparation of the patient, generation of x-radiation, and film processing and interpretation.

Orbitale (Or): In cephalometric radiography, the lowest point on the contour of the bony orbit.

Osteitis: A bone inflammation. In radiography, the term refers to changes in bone density resulting from disease, trauma, or infection. In rarefying osteitis the bone appears more radiolucent, whereas in condensing osteitis, the bone structures appear more radiopaque.

Osteomyelitis: An acute or chronic inflammation of the bone or bone marrow, which may sometimes be visible on radiographs.

Overlapping: A term used in radiography to refer to a distortion of the tooth image in which the structures of one tooth are superimposed over the structures of the adjacent tooth. This is most often caused by faulty horizontal angulation of the central beam.

Oxidation: In dental radiography, the process during which the chemicals of the developing and fixing solutions combine with oxygen and lose their strength.

Oxidizing Agent: Any substance that produces oxidation in another substance.

Panoramic Radiography: Radiographic procedures with a special purpose x-ray machine that uses a fixed position of the x-ray source, object, and film to produce a radiograph of the entire dentition and surrounding structures on a single film.

Parallax: In photography, a condition in which the viewing lens shows less than the photographer sees.

Paralleling Technique (Long-Cone Technique or Right-Angle Technique): In radiography, an intraoral exposure technique that requires a biteblock or some type of film holder to hold the film packet parallel to the teeth while the central beam of radiation is directed perpendicularly (at right angles) toward the teeth and the film.

Particulate Radiation: (See **Corpuscular Radiation.**)

Pedodontic Film: The smaller sizes of film packets commonly used for radiographs of children's teeth.

Penumbra: In radiography, a shadow or fuzzy outline around the image. Often caused by motion of the patient or tube head during exposure.

Periapical Radiograph: A radiograph that shows completely the entire tooth or teeth in a given dental region, and also shows all or parts of the adjacent tissues and oral structures.

Personnel Monitoring: The occasional or routine measuring of the amount of radiation to which a person working around radiation has been exposed during a given period of time. This is most often accomplished by wearing a film badge or a pocket dosimeter.

Phantom (Dexter): In dental radiography, a device the size and shape of the head and usually containing parts of the skull and all of the teeth. This is covered with plastic and other materials that resemble the lips, cheeks, tongue, and other facial structures. These materials scatter x-radiation in approximately the same ways as the tissues of the body do. The jaws are opened and closed by means of mechanical spring-type devices to enable the student to position and expose films in lieu of patients,

Phosphors: Fluorescent crystals, usually calcium tungstate, used in the emulsion that coats the intensifying screens. These give off light when subjected to radiation.

Photon (X-ray Photon): A quantum of light energy, analogous to the electron. X-rays are believed to be minute bundles of pure energy. These x-ray photons are often referred to as "bullets of energy."

PID: (See **Position Indicating Device** or **Cone**.)

Plane: In dental radiography, a level surface or a straight line connecting two anatomic landmarks.

Pocket Dosimeter: A small personnel monitoring device that resembles a fountain pen in size and can be clipped to the garment to measure radiation received. (See **Dosimeter**.)

Pogonion (Pg or Pog): In cephalometric radiography, the most anterior prominent point on the contour of the chin.

Point of Entry: The spot on the surface of the face toward which the central beam of radiation is directed when making intraoral exposures.

Polychromatic: A term from the Greek meaning having many colors. This term is used in dental radiography to describe the x-ray beam that is composed of many wavelengths of different intensity.

Porion (P): In cephalometric radiography, the midpoint on the upper edge of the external auditory meatus (acoustic meatus).

Port: (See **Aperture**.)

Position Indicating Device (PID, Cone): Any device attached to the tube head at the aperture to direct the useful beam of radiation. It can be long or short, cylindrical or rectangular, and open or closed and pointed at the tip.

Positive Angulation (Positive Vertical Angulation or Plus Angulation): Angulation achieved by pointing the tip or end of the PID downward from a horizontal plane. In the bisecting technique, positive angulation is used to make all maxillary and interproximal exposures.

Positive Ion: An ion that has a positive electric charge. (See **Ion**.)

Potential: In radiography and electricity, the difference in relative voltage or amount of electric pressure between the negative and positive electrodes.

Preservative: In radiography and photography, one of the chemicals (sodium sulfite) used in both the developer and fixer solutions to slow down the rapid rate of oxidation and prevent spoilage of the solution.

Primary Beam (Primary Radiation or Useful Beam): The original undeflected useful beam of radiation that emanates at the focal spot of the x-ray tube and emerges through the aperture of the tube head.

Primary Protective Barrier: A barrier sufficient to attenuate the useful beam to the required degree.

Processing Tank: A metal or hard rubber receptable divided into compartments for developer solution, water rinse, and fixer solution, and used to process radiographs.

Profile Radiographs (Lateral Headplates): Radiographs that record the shadow images of the soft tissues forming the facial curves and the features of the profile, and those forming the tongue and palate of the oral cavity. They are used to indicate the facial contours and to indicate the relationship of the soft to the bony tissues.

Protection Survey: An evaluation of the radiation hazards incidental to the production, use, or existence of sources of radiation under a specific set of conditions.

Protective Apron: An apron made of radiation-absorbing material (lead equivalent), used to protect the patient from unnecessary radiation exposure. (See **Lead Protective Apron**.)

Protective Barrier: A barrier of radiation absorbing materials, used to reduce radiation exposure. (See **Primary Protective Barrier** and **Secondary Protective Barrier**.)

Protective Tube Housing (Diagnostic Tube Housing): An x-ray tube housing so constructed that the leakage radiation measured at a distance of one meter from the target does not exceed 100 millirems in an hour when the tube is operated at its maximum continuous rated current for the maximum rated tube potential.

Qualified Expert: In dental radiation monitoring terminology, a person having the knowledge and training to measure ionizing radiation, to evaluate safety techniques, and to advise regarding radiation protection needs of dental x-ray installations.

Quantum: In the quantum theory, an elemental unit of energy. The theory holds that energy is not absorbed or radiated continuously but discontinuously in definite units called quanta.

Rad: A special unit of absorbed dose equal to 100 ergs per gram of tissue. For x-radiation, the rad is numerically the same as the roentgen.

Radiation: The emission and propagation of energy through space or through a material medium in the form of electromagnetic waves, corpuscular emissions such as alpha and beta particles, or rays of mixed and unknown types such as cosmic rays. Most radiations used in dentistry are capable of producing ions directly or indirectly by interaction with matter.

Radiation Field: The region in which energy is being propagated.

Radiation Hazard: The risk of exposure to radiation in an area where x-ray equipment is operating or where radioactive material is stored. Any uncontrolled source of radiation presents a potential danger.

Radiation Hygiene: Methods of protecting persons from accidental injury from exposure to radiation. Also includes techniques used to reduce and control the amounts of radiation used in medical and dental installations.

Radiation Monitoring: (See **Monitoring, Area Monitoring,** and **Personnel Monitoring.**)

Radiation Protection Supervisor: The person directly responsible for radiation protection and safety measures. In dental offices it is usually the dentist.

Radiation Protection Survey: In dentistry, an evaluation of the radiation safety in and around a dental office.

Radiator: A large mass of copper just outside the x-ray tube and connected to the anode terminal. The radiator functions to carry off the excess heat produced in the energy exchange that takes place when the electrons of the cathode stream are converted into about 1 percent x-rays and 99 percent heat. The copper of the radiator conducts the heat away from the target and cools the tube.

Radioactivity: The process whereby certain unstable elements undergo spontaneous disintegration (decay). The process is accompanied by emissions of one or more types of radiation and generally results in the formation of a new isotope.

Radiograph: An image produced on photosensitive film by exposing the film to x-rays and then developing the film so that a negative is produced. Also called an x-ray film, radiogram, roentgenogram, or roentgenograph.

Radiographer: Person who operates x-ray machine. (See **Operator.**)

Radiographic Fog: A darkening or clouding of the radiographic film image caused by exposure of the film to stray radiation during storage or by failure to protect the film from radiation while other exposures are made.

Radiography (Roentgenography): Generating and applying x-radiation to film sensitized for the purpose of making shadow pictures.

Radiolucent: That portion of the processed radiograph that is dark because the exposed structures lack density; or a subject that permits the passage of x-rays with little or no resistance.

Radiopaque: That portion of the radiographic film that appears light; or a subject that resists the passage of radiation.

Radioresistant: A substance or tissue that is not easily injured by ionizing radiation.

Radiosensitive: A substance or tissue that is relatively susceptible to injury by ionizing radiation.

Rarefaction: The state of being or becoming less dense, usually as a result of some disease process, indicated by radiolucent areas in the bone structures shown on radiographs.

Rectification: In radiography, the unidirectional current inside the x-ray tube from the cathode to the anode.

Rectifier: A device within the vacuum tube for converting the alternating to direct current.

Reducer: A chemical capable of bringing a salt into its metallic state by removing the nonmetallic elements.

Reduction: In dental radiography, a process in which an over-exposed or overdeveloped radiograph is placed in a reducing solution. This lightens the radiographic image by removing one layer of metallic silver at a time from the film surface.

Rem: The unit of dose equivalent. For radiation protection purposes, the number of rems of x-rays may be considered equal to the number of rads or the number of roentgens.

Restrainer: In radiography, the potassium bromide in the developer solution. It slows down the action of the elon and hydroquinine in the developer and inhibits the tendency of the solution to chemically fog the films.

Reticulation: Cracking of the film emulsion caused by a large temperature difference between the developer and the rinse water.

Right Angle Technique: (See **Paralleling Technique**.)

Roentgen (R): The unit of exposure to radiation. This is the exposure required to produce in air 2.58 times 10^4 (to the fourth power) coulomb of ions of either sign per kilogram of air. A simpler definition of the roentgen is that it is the amount of x or gamma radiation required to ionize one cc. of air at standard conditions of pressure and temperature.

Roentgenogram: (See **Radiograph**.)

Roentgenograph: (See **Radiograph**.)

Roentgenographer: (See **Radiographer** or **Operator**.)

Roentgenology (Radiology): The study and use of the roentgen ray in its application to dentistry and medicine.

Roentgenolucent: (See **Radiolucent**.)

Roentgenopaque: (See **Radiopaque**.)

Roentgen Ray (X-Ray): The radiant energy of short wavelength discovered by Wilhelm Konrad Roentgen in Germany in 1895 and designated as x-ray by him. This form of radiant energy has the power to penetrate substances that are ordinarily opaque, and to record shadow images on photographic film. The term roentgen ray is more technical than the more commonly used term x-ray.

Rule of Isometry: A geometric theorem which states that two triangles with two equal angles and a common side are equal triangles.

The application of this theorem to the bisecting technique was first suggested by Cieszynski in 1907 (Cieszynski's Law).

Safelight: A special type of filtered light that can be left burning in the darkroom while films are processed. The safelight rays do not affect the film emulsion unless the filter is defective, too close to the film being exposed, or allowed to shine on the unprocessed film for too long.

Scatter Radiation: Radiation that has been deflected from its path by impact during its passage through matter. This form of secondary radiation is emitted or deflected in all directions by the tissues of the patient's head during exposure to x-radiation.

Scintillation Counter: An area monitoring device containing a photoelectric cell that helps to measure the flashes of visible light emitted when the radiation that bombards certain salt crystals causes them to fluoresce.

Screen Film: A type of extraoral film for use in cassettes with intensifying screens. This film has an emulsión that is more sensitive to the blue and violet lights, emitted when the radiation strikes the phosphors in the intensifying screens, than to the x-radiation.

Secondary Protective Barrier: A barrier sufficient to attenuate stray radiation to the required degree.

Secondary Radiation: The radiation given off by any matter irradiated with x-rays. Radiation that results from the interaction of the primary beam, the PID, air, or human tissues. This is a new form of radiation that is created at the instant the primary beam interacts with matter and gives off some of its energy, forming new and less powerful wavelengths. This is often referred to as scatter radiation.

Selective Reduction: A chemical change that takes place within the film emulsion during development. During this change, the nonmetallic elements are separated from the silver halide of the exposed grains, leaving a coating of metallic silver on the film emulsion while the bromide is removed. The process is called selective because the unexposed grains are not reduced.

Self-Induction: An electrical term referring to the ability of a single coil in an autotransformer to vary the current and potential in a near by circuit.

Self-Rectification: In radiography, the ability of the x-ray machine to produce x-rays only during that portion of the alternating current cycle when the cathode has a negative and the anode has a positive charge.

Sensitivity: (See **Emulsion Speed.**)

Shells: (See **Energy Levels.**)

Shield (Shielding): A protective barrier of structural materials.

Short Scale Contrast: The variations in contrast, with few shades of gray as when the differences between blacks and whites on the radiograph are great. Fewer shades are produced when low kilovoltage is used.

Skin Dose: (See **Entrance Dose.**)

Soft Radiation: Rays of low energy and long wavelengths that have little penetrating power. These have no value in producing dental radiographs and are removed from the polychromatic beam by filtration.

Somatic Cells: All body cells except the reproductive cells.

Somatic Effects: In radiography, the effect of radiation on all body cells except the reproductive cells, especially the effect on the blood, the soft muscular tissues and the bone.

Source: In radiography, the place where the x-ray photons originate. This is the focal spot on the target of the anode inside the x-ray tube.

Source-Film Distance: (See **Target-Film Distance.**)

Source-Surface Distance (Source-Skin Distance, Target-Skin Distance or Target-Surface Distance): The distance measured along the path of the central ray from the center of the focal spot (front surface of the target) to the surface of the skin or irradiated object.

Stray Radiation: The sum of the leakage and scattered radiation; radiation that emanates from parts of the tube other than the focal spot.

Structural Shielding: The protection afforded by building materials, such as the thickness of a stucco wall.

Subject Contrast: The area-to-area difference in density in a radiograph caused by the differing thicknesses of the tissues or the object radiographed.

Surface Dose: The amount of radiation at the skin surface measured in rems.

Syndrome: A group of symptoms that together characterize a disease or lesion.

Target: The small block of tungsten imbedded in the face of the anode, bombarded by the electrons streaming toward it from the cathode. The focal spot is located on the target.

Target-Film Distance (Source-Film Distance or Focus-Film Distance): The distance between the focal spot on the target and the recording plane of the film. Generally, this distance is 8 inches when the bisecting technique is used and 16 or more inches for the paralleling technique.

Target-Object Distance (Source-Object Distance or Focus-Object Distance): The distance between the target on the anode in the x-ray tube and the object being radiographed.

Target-Surface Distance (Source-Surface Distance): The distance between the target and the surface of the object being radiographed.

Temporomandibular Joint Radiograph (TMJ Radiograph): An extraoral film used to show in profile the articulation of the head of the mandibular condyle with the glenoid fossa of the temporal bone and the surrounding structures.

Thermionic Emission: The release of electrons when a material such as tungsten is heated to incandescence; specifically, the boiling off of electrons from the cathode filament in the x-ray tube when electric current is passed through it.

Threshold Exposure: The minimum exposure that will produce a detectable degree of any given effect.

Timer: A mechanical, electrical, or electronic device that can be set to predetermine the duration of the interval that the current flows through the x-ray machine to produce x-rays.

Topographical Technique: A method used in occlusal radiography, in which the rules of bisecting are followed and the radiation beam is directed through the apices of the teeth perpendicularly toward the bisector. Because a larger area is involved and it is not always possible to use the most favorable vertical angulation, the images of the teeth generally appear longer than on a periapical radiograph of the same area.

Total Filtration: The combination of the inherent and added filtration in an x-ray machine. Many states require a total filtration of 2.5 mm. of aluminum equivalent for x-ray machines operating at above 70 kVp.

Tragus-Ala Line (Ala-Tragus Line): An imaginary plane or line from the tragus of the ear (the cartilagenous projection in front of the acoustic meatus of the ear) and the ala of the nose (a winglike projection at the side of the nose). This plane is important in positioning the patient's head correctly in the bisecting technique.

Transformer: One of several types of electrical devices capable of increasing or decreasing the voltage of an alternating current by mutual induction between primary and secondary coils or windings on cores of metal. (See **High-Voltage Transformer** and **Low-Voltage Transformer**.)

Trough: The low spot in the wave form; the opposite of the crest of the wave.

Tube Head: The protective metal covering that contains the x-ray tube, the tube housing, the transformers, and insulating oil. It forms the core of the most essential components of the x-ray machine and is attached to the flexible extension arm by a yoke. The PID attaches to the tube head at the aperture.

Tube Side: A term used to describe the side of the film packet or the exposure holder or cassette that must be positioned facing the source of x-rays coming from the tube.

Tungsten (Wolfram): An element with an atomic number of 74. Owing to its high melting point, this metal is extremely suitable to use as the cathode filament and as the anode target in the production of x-rays.

Useful Beam (Useful Radiation): That part of the primary beam that is permitted to emerge from the housing of the tube and is limited by the aperture, filters, collimeter diaphragm or other collimating device such as a lead-lined PID.

Vertical Angulation: The direction of the central beam in an up or down direction achieved by directing the tip of the PID upward or downward. (See **Negative Angulation** and **Positive Angulation**.)

Viewer (View Box or Illuminator): A device for concentration or reflecting light; generally, a lamp behind an opaque glass used for viewing radiographs.

Volt: A unit of electromotive force or potential that is sufficient to cause a current of one ampere to flow through a resistance of one ohm.

Voltage: Electrical pressure or force that drives the electric current through the circuit of the x-ray machine. (See **Kilovolt** and **Kilovolt Peak**.)

Voltmeter: A device for measuring the electromotive force (the difference in potential or voltage) across the x-ray tube.

Wavelength: In radiography, the length in Angstrom units of the electromagnetic radiations produced in the x-ray machine.

Wetting Agent: A chemical preparation similar to a detergent that reduces the surface tension of film. A small amount may be added to the developer or the final rinse water to facilitate development and drying of the radiograph.

Window: In radiography, the thin wall of glass in an x-ray tube opposite the focal spot. The primary x-ray beam leaves the tube through this thin area of the tube envelope.

Workload: In radiography, the total time that the x-ray machine is used, expressed in milliampere seconds per week.

X-Ray: (See **Roentgen Ray.**)

X-Ray Film: (See **Radiograph or Film Packet.**)

X-Ray Film Hanger: Mechanical devices for holding intraoral and extraoral film in the processing solutions and while drying.

X-Ray Timer: A clock-like device that can be set for the intervals required in processing. It is activated by a lever and rings when the interval has elapsed. Can be set in ¼-second increments.

Yoke: The curved portion of the x-ray machine that can revolve 360 degrees horizontally where it is connected to the extension arm. The tube head is suspended within the yoke and can be rotated vertically within it.

Zero Angulation (Zero Vertical Angulation): Angulation achieved by directing the tip of the PID so that the entire PID is parallel with the plane of the floor. When directed in this manner, the central beam travels parallel with the plane of the floor. (See **Negative Angulation** and **Positive Angulation.**)

index